Canary In A Coal Mine

Canary In A Coal Mine

by

B. Carolyn Knight

Aristan Press

Library of Congress Catalog Card Number 84-71899
ISBN 0-931407-00-1

Cover by Barna Hudson Design
Aristan Press
Post Office Box 395
Placentia, California 92670

Dedicated with love
and heartfelt thanks
to my life-savers
Sally, Ros and Vick

Foreword

Medicine today is a highly technical field, where doctor and patient alike are blinded by a blizzard of information. Since the physician's time is often taken up in the attempt to verify whether or not the patient fits into a particular category, he is unable to spend as much time as he would like discovering the details of the patient's lifestyle, symptoms and medical problems. With the increasing expense and complexity of medicine, the burden of health will increasingly be shared by the patient. Where allergy is concerned, it is even more important for the patient to accept an active role—the doctor explaining the principles and what to look for and the patient assuming the part of a Sherlock Holmes by supplying the doctor with as much information as possible about his or her reactions.

Carolyn Knight's story indicates how valuable it is to have a patient well-educated about her own disease. In Carolyn's case, an informed attitude and a willing acceptance of responsibility for her own well-being resulted in a breakthrough which will be of benefit to many others.

Canary in a Coal Mine contains a message for doctors and patients alike: a receptive physician and an alert patient working together can add a new dimension to the field of health.

—Leo H. Cummins, M.D.

President
Orange County Society
for Allergy and Clinical Immunology
Past President
Los Angeles County Society
for Allergy and Clinical Immunology

During the many years I've suffered from asthma and throughout the months of research I undertook to discover its cause, I was encouraged by friends, doctors and other allergy sufferers to share my story. Though hesitant to do so at first, I finally realized that putting my plight in book form could serve several purposes. It could help ease the shame and suffering of other adult asthmatics who have been told for years that their asthma is nothing more than a psychosomatic condition. It could encourage others with wheezes, sniffles, itches and watery eyes to search themselves for the reasons behind their maladies. It could inspire patients to take more of a responsibility for their own health. And, probably more importantly, it could sound an alarm to the entire population about the indiscriminate use of chemicals in our nation's food supply.

My thanks to all who encouraged me. To my family, who listened, cried and laughed with me during the cathartic project. To Joan Dial, who convinced me that my story did belong in a book. To the staff at Scripps Clinic and Research Foundation for its support and understanding. And to Dr. Leo Cummins for his friendship and assistance.

All of the events in the book are true and the tests documented. However, the names of the physicians have been changed.

—B.C.K.

1

Gasping for breath, I made my way into the ladies' room and sought refuge in one of the cramped metal cubicles. The small quarters were claustrophobic, and the overhead fan seemed to be robbing the room of oxygen rather than circulating it. I pulled up my skirt, rolled down my pantyhose and fumbled in my purse for the small vial of adrenalin and the syringe I kept there. My hands were shaking, and my breathing was becoming even more labored as I pinched the skin of my thigh with my left hand and plunged the needle into my leg. Sitting back on the stool, I leaned my head against the hard partition and prayed that the injection would take effect before I lost consciousness.

After eleven years I should be getting used to these episodes. But how does one become accustomed to the terror of respiratory arrest and the knowledge that death can occur in minutes if proper medical care is not taken?

As the adrenalin surged through my body, putting all my cells on alert, I began to feel my lungs expand and welcomed a long, deep breath.

Thank God. I stood up to straighten my clothes, left the unattractive sanctuary of the stall and walked out to face the large mirror, splattered with water stains from careless hands. I pulled a brush through my unruly brown curls and stared at my reflection, looking for signs of a debilitating illness. There were none. My color was good and my dark eyes sparkled, thanks to the effects of the miracle drug I carried in my handbag.

Fight or flight. I remembered the definition of adrenalin learned from a high school biology teacher and thought how the phrase could also be applied to my life.

How often I had felt like doing battle with this disabling disease.

And how often I'd felt like running away from it all since illness had taken control of my life in 1971 . . . .

"Mommy?" Kathy took a tentative step into my bedroom.

"I'm awake, honey." I held out my hand to my eight-year-old daughter, beckoning her to my side. "Mommy can't get up this morning, Trink . . . Can you be my big helper . . . and get yourself . . . and your little sister . . . ready for school?"

"Can't you breathe very well today, Mommy?" Kathy's big brown eyes began to fill with tears as she heard the all too familiar wheezing coming from deep within me. "Maybe Daddy can come home from work to take care of you."

"Don't worry . . . I'm seeing the doctor today . . . and I'll be all better . . . by the time you girls . . . get home from school."

My shortness of breath made it difficult for me to speak, but I tried to calm my daughter with my words.

"Now you get dressed . . . and choose something pretty for Meri to wear . . . and a pair of socks that match . . . and bring them to me . . . I'll help her get ready . . . while you fix some cereal for the two of you . . . okay?"

Lying back against the pillow, I gazed out the bedroom window and watched the delicate branches of the California pepper tree blowing in the misty morning breeze. My young husband, Jerry, and I had moved to the picturesque community of Huntington Beach four years before. We loved the nearness of the ocean and the tangy smell of the salt water. We had watched our two toddlers grow into bright and beautiful school girls and still marveled at our good fortune in finding a house we could afford in such an ideal setting. The beach was less than a mile away, and we loved to bicycle there on warm summer evenings to let the girls play in the sand or to fly kites in the gentle sea breezes.

I closed my eyes and sighed. Once again I was overwhelmed as I thought of the changes that had occurred in my life in the last few months. Though I had been prone to bouts of bronchitis as a child and teenager, I'd always considered myself a healthy person. Oh, sure, there were frequent nights of wheezing since our move to the beach area. But weak lungs ran in the family, and I blamed the damp, foggy air. Until six months ago, I had awakened each morning looking forward to a day brimming with activity. Besides caring for the house and children, I kept busy serving as a deaconess and as chairman of the wedding committee at our church, working as a volunteer for the Braille Institute and spearheading the Girl Scout functions in which my daughters were involved. Most importantly to me, I had been taking 12 units at the local college and working toward my life-long goal of a bachelor of arts degree.

Now, except for continuing with just one class—for I refused to withdraw from school completely—it was all I could do to perform even the most simple of tasks.

Long nights of laboring for each breath, coughing spells that left me choking and exhausted, mornings when I was completely winded from merely making the beds, days that I couldn't walk across the living room to answer the phone because it required too much breath to do so—these were the ways I had to describe my life now.

My God, I was only 27-years-old, and I felt like an invalid at least twice that age.

Later, driving to the internist's office, I tried to push away the frightening thoughts that had been plaguing me since the most recent series of tests had begun two weeks before.

Could I have tuberculosis?

Emphysema?

Even lung cancer was a possibility, I feared, pulling into the parking lot of the medical center and shivering at the thought. I was early, but I knew it would take me twice as long as it once had to walk the distance from the car to the building and then make my way to the seventh floor office.

After peering into my ears and throat, thumping me on the back and listening to my chest with his stethoscope, Dr. Adkins asked me to step into his office. I sat in the straight-backed chair, biting my lower lip while the doctor rummaged through some papers and buzzed his nurse to bring in the lecture notes he'd need before addressing a meeting that evening.

I'd begun to wonder if he'd forgotten I was there when, finally, he swiveled in his large upholstered chair and turned his attention to me.

"Carolyn, it looks as if your problems are being caused by asthma."

I stared at him, unable to speak and incredulous over the diagnosis. Conflicting thoughts went through my mind. Asthma is a psychosomatic illness, one that can be turned on and off. It's the ploy of a willful child wanting his own way. Surely it couldn't describe my failing health. He must be mistaken.

Dazed, I tried to concentrate on the doctor's words.

"Adult-onset asthma is usually a chronic condition—one you'll just have to learn to live with." He went on in a matter-of-fact tone. "There is no cure, but we'll do our best to control it through medication."

Dr. Adkins stood up, as if to dismiss me and any questions I might have.

Accepting the prescription form he handed me, I left his office as quickly as my breathlessness would allow. Being chronically ill just didn't fit into my plans. I fought back tears as the elevator swooshed toward the lobby. I'll find another doctor. Maybe an allergist could help. Or a pulmonary specialist. I'll even give a faith healer a try, I thought, vowing to find an answer, a drug, a miracle—anything that would restore my former good health.

2

I pushed open the door of the converted yellow house that was Dr. Whitmore's office and was welcomed by a chorus of greetings.

"Hi, Carolyn."

"How's it going?"

"Hey, you really sneaked up on us today. We can usually hear you wheezing a mile away."

In the year that I had been coming to the allergist's office, the nurses and I had become quite friendly, and I was even able to call many of the other patients by name, because we saw each other so often during our twice-weekly visits.

I walked into the brightly wallpapered injection room and rolled up my sleeve, calculating that this was the 104th time I had done so. My main activities this past year have been driving to and from doctors' offices, popping pills and getting shots, I thought. But I shouldn't complain. I *was* feeling better. In fact, after leaving the office today, I was going to meet my sister, Sally, and our Aunt Margaret for lunch.

I offered my pin-pricked upper arm to the nurse and barely winced as the needle pierced my skin. Testing I had undergone a year ago had discovered a slight allergy to mold, but attempts to immunize me against the fungus had failed. Dr. Whitmore now theorized that I was allergic to the bacteria in my own body, and for the past eight weeks I had been receiving injections from a special serum he had concocted from my own body juices—complete with its resident bacteria and germs.

My first few months as Dr. Whitmore's patient had not been easy ones. The allergist had made it clear from the beginning that he'd treat my asthma, but wouldn't take care of me when I was sick for any other reason.

At that time I was plagued by frequent infections, which adversely affected—if not caused—my shortness of breath, and I was unable to distinguish one from another.

There were many times that I'd enter Dr. Whitmore's office, barely able to walk, and he'd refuse to see me.

"Carolyn, I've told you not to come in when you're sick," he'd scold me as if I were a naughty child. "Do you want to infect all of my other patients?"

Feeling properly chastised and even stupid for not being able to determine an illness caused by infection from a common everyday asthma attack, I dutifully traveled between my allergist and my internist, taking pills and advice from Dr. Whitmore one week and from Dr. Adkins the next.

At one point I was so frustrated and sick that I wished I could find a doctor who would take a more holistic approach. But how does a person start all over again to find another physician? Both of mine had come highly recommended as "the best in their fields," and the idea of being without them while I searched for someone else to care for me was a frightening one.

Luckily my illnesses had been few throughout the summer months, and Dr. Whitmore had not had to admonish me for quite some time. Maybe my doctors were right in their approach after all. I'd certainly been under much better control recently.

Within 10 minutes of my arrival, I was on my way back out the door, amid jokes from the nurses that I might as well move in and save myself the long drives back and forth.

Maneuvering my car onto the nearby freeway and into the flow of traffic, I headed for Lakewood and my luncheon date and allowed my mind to reminisce over the past year's events.

After my initial reaction to the diagnosis of asthma, I had become more rational as the prescribed medication allowed me to lead a more normal life. My respiratory condition was still severe, however, robbing me of my sleep, affecting my ability to take part in physical activities and causing me to eliminate many of the outside interests in which I'd been involved. I required daily cortisone to control my shortness of breath, in addition to bronchodilators and inhalation therapy, but I *was* improving. And with both Dr. Adkins and Dr. Whitmore working on my case, my hopes were high.

I had not yet added a faith healer to my growing list of doctors, but I had seen a psychologist. I had heard so often that asthma stemmed from emotional disorders, and I had almost hoped it did—for then I could apply the philosophy of mind over matter and be responsible for my own cure.

I had spent days in the college library, poring over medical texts to uncover the causes of asthma and attempting to apply them to my own life. Because the disease defied medical interpretation, I found that physicians for years had tended to blame emotional causes. Even Hippocrates said that, "the asthmatic must guard against anger."

The psychosomatic theory was given further credence by physician Rene Laennec, who invented the stethoscope. Because the French doctor could find no organic reason for asthma with his new instrument, he concluded in 1819 that the disease could be attributed to "mental emotion."

I had been especially intrigued by the writings of Joseph Bicknell Chapin, an American doctor who wrote in 1843 that a nervous temperament and irritability invited asthma. Completely perplexed by the disease, he wrote, "What will almost universally relieve one case, will as assuredly induce a paroxysm in another. Ordinarily the air of the low situations is more congenial than mountain breezes . . . .Some suffer in a certain room, but are immediately relieved if removed to an opposite room in the same house. One cannot sleep or rest in one street or lane, but slumbers quietly if removed to another part of the same village or city."

I sighed. Asthma was puzzling and confusing. No wonder it was considered psychosomatic.

On the chance that my own disease might have emotional roots, I had spent many hours figuratively putting my life under a microscope, first taking a long, hard look at my marriage. It could hardly be described as the "happily ever after" I had expected as a starry-eyed teenage wife, but was I miserable enough that my unhappiness would manifest itself in disease? I thought not. Perhaps causing me more grief at the time was the fact that my best friend and confidante was moving and, although she'd only be two hours away, our daily get-togethers and constant phone calls would have to cease. Could my sadness over losing my dear friend be contributing to my dilemma? Not too likely for an independent sort such as I. And, as trivial as it would sound to most, I had just received a "C" in a college course—the first "low" grade I had ever gotten in my life. Was the importance I placed on my education coupled with the humiliation I felt at receiving a mere average grade causing my health to deteriorate? I doubted it. Yet wanting to do all I could to control my condition and my life, I had begun seeing Dr. Kingsley.

After probing into my childhood, discussing sibling rivalry and investigating my relationship with my parents, the $50 an hour psychologist had proclaimed my asthma was "caused by an unresolved conflict with the female parent."

Now, I had come across that theory in my library research and had handily rejected it. I couldn't believe I'd paid a bearded, myopic shrink more than $500 to come up with this time-worn philosophy. For that amount of money he could have been more creative.

Oh, sure, Mom and I had had our problems while I was growing up—what teenager and her mother hadn't? But now that I was a mother myself, she and I had a wonderful loving relationship. How absurd that a psychologist would think I had developed asthma as a result of my mother not allowing me to shave my legs until I was 15—or because I still resented having to be home from dates earlier than any of my friends.

So much for the psychosomatic theory, I thought as I made a turn into the parking lot of the restaurant where I had agreed to meet my aunt and sister.

I saw them immediately as I walked into the coffee shop—tall, blonde Sally talking animatedly to a smiling Aunt Margaret. A close family, we greeted each other lovingly. My aunt squeezed my hand, "You look so well today, sweetheart." I assured her that was just the way I felt, too.

We analyzed the plastic-coated menus, discussing the culinary pros and cons of each item before all deciding to order the chef's salad. We carried on a lively conversation until our lunches arrived and then all quieted for a time to savor the thin slices of ham, turkey and cheese atop a bed of fresh lettuce.

After several bites, I noticed that the palms of my hands and the soles of my feet were beginning to itch. How odd, I thought, trying to ignore the extremely uncomfortable feeling. Within minutes, however, the sensations within my body could no longer be disregarded. Besides the increased itching of my hands and feet, my lungs felt almost paralyzed, and I was having great difficulty drawing in any air.

"Sis, all of a sudden . . . I can't breathe," I said, finding it hard to speak.

Turning from a discussion with Aunt Margaret about the upcoming election, Sally took one look at me and jumped up from the booth. She grabbed my arm and helped me scoot out from behind the table, leading me outside.

"Sit down," she said, pointing to the corner of a brick planter surrounding the restaurant. "I'll get the car."

Obediently I took her advice and attempted to still the feeling of panic rising in me as I struggled for each breath. I rubbed my hands on the rough surface of the bricks and wriggled my toes inside my shoes, trying to alleviate the intense itching. Automatically my chin jutted forward as my oxygen-starved body made an effort to open its airways. I could feel my nostrils flaring in yet another of my body's reactions to extreme shortness of breath.

I was hardly aware of Sally's blue Volkswagen bug pulling up alongside me, as I continued to sit on the planter.

"Damn it, *get in*," she ordered in an almost angry tone that masked her fear. But this time I was unable to respond to her command, so she shoved open her door and half carried me to the passenger side, managing to push me into the seat just as I lost consciousness.

As the scene was reconstructed for me later, Sally roared through the red light at the intersection with her hand held on the horn and pulled into the entrance of the small private hospital across the street. Screeching to a halt in front of the emergency ward, she looked at my gray lips, blue face and unseeing eyes and, thinking I could breathe easier if my tight jeans were unfastened, attempted to unzip my pants. Her nervousness impeded her ability to perform the simple task, however, and she gave up, deciding it was more important to get help.

Rushing through the door of the emergency room, Sally ran to the frosted window where the receptionist sat.

"I need help fast," she said, breathless herself from the stress of the situation.

"Fill out this form. We'll be with you as soon as we can."

"You don't understand. My sister is dying," Sally screamed.

The receptionist looked at Sally patronizingly, continuing to hold out the clipboard with the consent form attached.

Half crying and hysterical, Sally ran back to the car. If they see the shape Carolyn's in they'll have to help, she reasoned. Opening the passenger door, she attempted to lift me in her arms. Despite the extra strength she was unable to do more than lower the upper half of my body to the asphalt. She left me half in and half out of the car and once again ran through the glass doors of the hospital.

Ignoring the receptionist and pushing through the adjacent swinging doors, she bounded down the long, antiseptic corridor crying for help. A nurse, unable to understand my sister's distraught babbling, took her arm and began to lead her into an office.

"Come with me, dear," the woman said in a condesending voice. "Sit down in here and tell me what's wrong."

Roughly releasing herself from the nurse's grasp, Sally once again started down the hall, searching for help. She spotted a man in green surgical garb and dashed to his side. Struggling to make her words understood, she gasped, "She can't breathe. My sister's dying. Parking lot. Hurry."

Running with Sally back down the corridor, the doctor yelled to the nurse, "Code blue!" and sent the surprised woman hurrying for more help.

Once in the parking lot, the doctor pulled me none too gently from the car and at once began mouth-to-mouth resuscitation. As Sally stood helplessly over my prostrate body, she noticed that I had lost control of my bladder and, knowing that to be a sign of near-death, she again began to cry unconsolably. Rushing out the doors with resuscitation equipment, the emergency staff gathered around. While one doctor injected my vein with 1000 mg of cortisone, another thrust a tube down my throat and began a flow of pure oxygen into my lungs.

Convulsed with grief, Sally continued her panic-stricken cries.

"She's dying. My sister's dying. Please don't let her die. Please don't let her die."

Leading her away from the scene, a nurse attempted to calm my anguished sister. Engaging her in conversation to distract her, the nurse discovered that our aunt was still at the restaurant and offered to go get her.

By the time Aunt Margaret arrived at the hospital, I was stabilized and in the Intensive Care Unit. Watching my still unconscious form through the tiny window of the door leading into the ICU, Sally and Aunt Margaret hugged each other and prayed.

Four hours later, weakened and exhausted from my trauma, I opened my eyes.

"Welcome back," said a doctor, touching my cheek. As a nurse continued to monitor my vital signs, the doctor began to ask me questions. What was my name? Where did I live? Where had I been before being brought to the hospital?

God, I was tired, but I answered his queries slowly and apparently gave him the information he wanted. Walking outside the ward, he spoke to my husband and the other family members who had gathered in the small waiting room. Soon, through the thick insulated walls, I could hear shouts and cries.

But this time they were shouts and cries of happiness, as my loved ones loudly rejoiced that I had regained consciousness and that I had not been without oxygen long enough to cause brain damage.

3

Dr. Adkins, what happened to me?"

Fear had sent me hurrying back to my internist the minute I was released from the hospital, and now I once again faced him over the vastness of his mahogany desk. I felt small and vulnerable as I waited for an explanation of the frightening attack that had almost taken my life.

"The best we can determine is that you choked on a piece of lettuce."

Tears, so near the surface since my terrible ordeal, rushed to my eyes.

"No, that's not what happened. I'm sure I didn't choke."

The doctor smiled at me patiently and reached across his desk to pat my hand.

"Now, Carolyn, I know this has been a very emotional experience for you. I've spoken with the doctors who cared for you in the hospital and the only explanation they have is that you choked on your lunch."

As I again began to protest, the doctor stopped me.

"When a piece of food got lodged in your windpipe, you couldn't breathe. You panicked, and that triggered an asthma attack. The combination of the two was very serious indeed, but don't blow the episode out of proportion."

Though my mind vehemently denied the doctor's conclusion, I decided not to press the point. What was the use? Who was I to tell the doctor? Instead I meekly listened to Dr. Adkins' orders and accepted the fistful of prescriptions he handed me.

I stopped by the pharmacy on the way home and was appalled not only by the multitude of pills, drops and syrups I was to take daily, but also by their price. I wrote out a check for $127 and was thankful once again that we had a good insurance policy.

At home I unpacked my month's supply of medications and wondered aloud how I would ever keep track of them all. Some I was to take twice a day, some four times a day, some before meals and some on an empty stomach.

"Why don't you make a chart, Mommy, like the one you made for Kathy and me?"

Out of the mouth of babes.

I bent down and scooped up my six year old, hugging her close. "What a super idea, Meri. Your chart reminds you and your sister to brush your teeth and put your toys away, and my chart will remind me when to take my medicines."

"And, if you're a good girl and take all your pills, you can get a star for your chart just like we do."

How sweet and uncomplicated is the life of a child, I thought as I sent my daughter out to play and began to clean off a kitchen shelf too high to be reached by little hands.

I looked at each medicine bottle as I put it on the shelf and remembered Dr. Adkins' explanation for each. There was potassium iodide to thin mucus, suspended theophylline to keep my airways open, nose drops to keep me from developing upper-respiratory symptoms, antibiotics to take as prophylactics against infection, bronchodilators to keep my respiratory track unobstructed, cortisone to reduce inflammation, and phenobarbitol to counteract the shaking that the adrenalin-type drugs caused.

What a different person I'd become. I had never liked to take medicine and had even avoided "drugging" my body with aspirin in the past. Now I relied on my pills and potions like a junkie.

At least I was living in a modern age when the symptoms of asthma could be alleviated, I told myself as I continued to arrange my bottles and jars. I recently had checked out a book from the university library that discussed asthma cures of the past century and had been quite shocked at the treatments. Tortures would describe the crude procedures more accurately.

I closed my eyes and let my imagination take over. I pictured myself an asthmatic in 1840, feeling the first frightening signs of an impending attack . . . .

It's past midnight, and I hear the relentless winter wind batter the shutters outside my bedroom window. I cough in an attempt to clear my lungs. My chest begins to tighten, then rattle as the mucus increases in my constricted airways.

I leave the warmth of the four-poster bed, taking care not to awaken my snoring husband, and make my way downstairs and into the kitchen. Remembering my physician's advice, I pull the old metal tub into the center of the room and fill it with cold water. Not bothering to set the screen around the tub for privacy, I disrobe and plunge my body into the icy bath. I am laboring for each breath, and my skin breaks out in goose bumps. I shiver. My teeth chatter, and I hug myself as I force my body to remain in the freezing water for the recommended length of time. The muscles of my back and chest begin to ache as I desperately battle to draw in the fresh air my body craves.

The hoped-for relief does not come.

I grab the rounded sides of the over-sized wash basin and pull myself to my feet, now gasping frantically for each breath. My movements have alerted my family and, seeing my pale face and bluish lips, my husband rushes out of the house to fetch the doctor. By the time he arrives, my daughters have helped me slip on my robe and have guided me to the horsehair davenport in the parlor. I could not have climbed the stairs to my bedroom.

Quickly examining me, the doctor decides to rely on the standard treatment of the day for asthmatics.

"We must make her vomit," he tells my family, sending them scurrying for towels and a large basin.

Reaching into his black bag, he pulls out a small bottle and hesitates for a moment as he tries to decide whether to use ipecac or a concoction made of garlic, mustard and "vinegar of squills," a dried plant commonly employed as a rat poison.

I am now so weak that the doctor must hold my head as I sip the foul-tasting medicinal drink. My stomach reacts on cue, and my terrible retching purges my body of all except my worsening asthma.

The doctor rushes back to his grip and uncaps a bottle of chloroform, encouraging me to breathe deeply. He has found that the fragrant fumes of the colorless liquid have a more positive effect than other inhalants of the day, such as burning nitrite paper or jimson weed. Tonight's attack, however, defies even this much-touted treatment, and the concerned doctor sends my older daughter into the kitchen to prepare a pot of strong black coffee, then reaches into the humidor on the small mahogany table and pulls out one of my husband's plump, brown cigars.

It has now been more than two hours since my horrifying attack began, and I am near exhaustion. My chest continues to heave and the sound of my wheezing fills the drafty room. The doctor hovers over me, coaxing me to draw as deeply as possible on the rounded tip of the cigar. The pungent nicotine makes my head spin, and my entire body feels weak and shaky. I break out in a cold sweat and swoon on the verge of unconsciousness. Suddenly a cup of coffee replaces the cigar at my lips, and I drink the strong, hot liquid.

Barely conscious, I fall back against the pillow of the couch once again and wait. The doctor has exhausted his list of remedies, and he and my family gather around my prostrate form watching for signs that I am receiving some relief.

My body shudders and I inhale the first deep breath I've been able to take in hours. My ordeal is over. I fall into a deep sleep, and my daughters cover me with a blanket, not willing to move me now that I am finally at rest. My husband walks the doctor to the door, thanks him and murmurs his goodbyes . . . .

I shook my head, ridding my mind of the fantasy. Perhaps my plight wasn't so bad after all. I looked at the neat row of medicine bottles now arranged on the top shelf of the cabinet. I'd rather take a ton of pills than smoke a cigar any day.

Dr. Adkins' other orders included the insistence that I drop most of my extracurricular activities. The one class a semester he begrudgingly allowed me to take was like a life-line to me. On the days I felt up to it, I arrived on the large, sprawling campus early enough to meet friends for lunch, and I especially enjoyed the fellowship and rap sessions that had always been such an important part of my life.

On a crisp fall day in 1972, I made arrangements to meet my friend, Ros Gibson, in the cafeteria. Choosing my favorite old standby of a chef's salad and iced tea, I sat at the long table delighting in the food and company. Half way through the meal, I realized that I was having increased difficulty breathing, but with a false sense of security brought about by the multitude of drugs I was taking, I didn't mention my problem to my friend and didn't realize I was in serious trouble until I left the cafeteria and began walking to class. I stumbled into the first restroom I could find and, oblivious to the chattering students combing their hair and applying make-up, I sat on the paper-strewn floor, leaned back against the wall and searched through my purse for the inhaler I used whenever I was short of breath.

The restroom door opened, and a middle-aged woman student walked in, looking at me curiously.

"Are you all right?" she asked me.

Not wanting to admit to her—or to myself—that I needed help, I nodded my head, still hoping that the inhalations I had just taken would soon begin to take effect.

Five minutes later I realized I had made a mistake by not telling the concerned stranger that I was ill. One o'clock classes had begun and the restroom was empty. I was alone, unable to walk, and the breathlessness I was experiencing, combined with the well-remembered sensations of itching hands and feet, were sure signs that I was once again heading toward a frightening episode like the one that had just months before almost taken my life.

Suddenly Ros's face loomed before me as she knelt beside me on the restroom floor. "Sue told me you were in here," she said, her soft southern drawl referring to the woman who had asked if I was all right. "Do you need to go to the hospital?"

Unable to talk because of lack of breath, I managed to convey my fear to my friend through panic-stricken eyes, and she squeezed my hands and reassured me that she'd be right back with help.

I remained on the floor, struggling for each breath of the artificial, pine-scented air and willed myself not to lose consciousness.

It seemed hours before Ros came back, leading a hesitant janitor into the women's restroom to carry me outside to a maintenance cart she had insisted he drive right to the door.

"We're going to take you to my car and then I'll drive you to the emergency ward," Ros said, once again squeezing my hand and hoping her calm manner would soothe me.

A crowd of gawking students began to gather as the custodian lifted me into the bright orange vehicle. It was only a two-seater so Ros ran alongside as we raced down the sidewalks of the campus on our way to the parking lot. I wanted the cart to hurry, yet the force of the wind caused by the high speed took my breath away even more, and I motioned for the man to slow down.

Winded herself from the long run, Ros found the superhuman strength needed to help me into the car.

"Don't worry. We're almost there," she said as we twisted through the parking area toward the exit. Despite her words, I could sense my friend's fear. The nearest hospital was more than two miles away on a large, busy street dotted with stop lights, and as I felt myself black out, I was certain we would not make it in time.

I awoke to the sounds of the hospital intercom and the sights of the steel gray equipment surrounding me. A hand smoothed my hair and I turned my head to see Ros leaning over the rail of the narrow hospital bed.

"Why'd you have to go do that? You had me scairt to death," she said, her Georgia upbringing evident in her accent. I gave her a groggy smile as she attempted to fill the silence and still our fears by making light of the way she had barreled toward the large Huntington Beach hospital with a blue passenger in tow.

My friend continued her one-sided conversation and refused to leave my side during the next hour while the emergency staff kept me under observation. Finally I was examined one last time and released, and as the nurse helped me to Ros's car, I leaned my head against the seat and closed my eyes so that I could be alone with my thoughts.

God, I was glad to be alive. But what was causing these violent asthma attacks? Would the doctors once again insist I had choked on food? I knew I would live my life in constant fear from now on, wondering when the next attack would occur.

4

Since medication had not protected me, I decided to turn once again to my allergist for help. Sitting on the edge of my seat in Dr. Whitmore's office the next week, I told him how I analyzed the situation.

"Both of my life-threatening attacks occurred in restaurants, so maybe the fumes from the kitchen irritated my lungs—or maybe I'm allergic to the institutional detergents they use on their glasses and silverware. It can't be the food, because I eat the same thing at home all the time without any problem."

Going on excitedly, I begged the allergist to help me play detective.

Dr. Whitmore held out his hand and, for a moment reminded me more of a traffic cop than a physician. "Hold on a minute, Carolyn, it's not as simple as you make it sound. We're sure now that the two episodes you've had recently are due to anaphylactic shock—extreme allergic reactions that lead to rapid loss of blood pressure and respiratory arrest."

He told me that whatever was causing my extreme response was something to which I was so intensely allergic that merely testing me with it could kill me.

"My advice to you," he concluded, "is to *go home* and *stay home* if you want to live long enough to see your children grow up."

Defeated, overcome by a sense of doom and feeling like a pawn who no longer had control over her own life, I went home and thought about my doctor's advice. For the greater part of two days, I alternated between fits of crying and bouts of rage directed at my own body. How dare it let me down like this? But I finally decided that, when I considered my priorities, at the top of the list were those two little girls who needed me so much. I withdrew from college the next day, resigned from my other commitments—and felt as if I were retiring from life.

Until now I had not realized that an allergy could be so devastating—that it could change a person's life forever. I'd always thought of allergy as a continually runny nose, a case of hives or itchy eyes. Yet now Dr. Whitmore was insisting that allergy was the cause of my asthma and its related episodes of anaphylactic shock.

The word allergy was always bantered about so freely. In fact, in the past I'd thought it was a term doctors used loosely to explain any illness for which they really couldn't find a cause. Now I wasn't so sure. What was an allergy anyway? Why is one person allergic and another not? Why did I suddenly become so deathly allergic at the age of 27? Why, why, why?

I decided to ask Dr. Whitmore during my next visit.

Unfortunately, my physician had neither the time nor the inclination to discuss the subject with me during my office call the following week.

"Carolyn, I'm sorry I don't have the time to explain all of this to you—you can see that the waiting room is full of patients I must see before lunch."

He turned and grabbed a brochure from the drawer of a small table in the corner of the room. Tossing it my way, he relinquished any responsibility for answering my question.

"You're an intelligent young woman. And since you no longer attend college, you can research allergy yourself. This pamphlet should help you understand it."

I stared at the door that he closed behind himself before I could even reply. I felt deflated, totally discounted and like a nonentity. To Dr. Whitmore I must be nothing more than a pair of diseased lungs—a misfunctioning machine that he had the duty to keep oiled and running.

I fought back tears as I took off the hospital gown I'd slipped on for Dr. Whitmore's cursory examination. I dressed quickly, gathered my purse and the brochure he'd given me and left the tiny room. Passing through the lobby on the way out, I glanced at the roomful of coughing, sneezing people. Perhaps I'd been too hasty to judge Dr. Whitmore. All of these fellow allergy-sufferers needed his attention, too. If he took time to answer every question he was asked during the day, he wouldn't be able to treat half the patients he did now. On the other hand, a smaller patient load *would* enable him to treat the *whole* person, not just his or her particular ailment.

But that wasn't my business, I supposed, and Dr. Whitmore was right about one thing. I did have the intelligence to research allergy on my own.

I hurried out of the office and set out for home—and the self-imposed exile that awaited me there.

Staying at home did have its rewards. I spent many hours of what child psychologists term "quality time" with my daughters and turned my creative instincts toward more domestic pursuits.

One day when I was in the middle of baking my own bread, Ros dropped by as she had so often since my doctor's blunt admonition several weeks before. Seeing me in a flour-smeared apron and with the white stuff smudged on my nose and cheek, Ros began to laugh.

"You look just like a housewife."

She hugged me, knowing that such a remark would have made both of us furious a couple of years before when women's liberation was "raising our consciousnesses." However, hours of talking with my dear friend and marathon discussions of my fears and frustrations had helped me begin to accept the new direction my life was taking.

"I brought you those books on allergy you wanted from the library," Ros said, dumping them on the kitchen table and walking over to the oven to see how my cinnamon bread was doing.

"Thanks," I said, thinking how wonderful Ros and my other friends had been to me during the time I'd been imprisoned in my own house. Besides running errands for me and doing my grocery shopping, they stopped by often to visit and lend their support. My husband, Jerry, had been understanding, too, as he discovered a new dimension to parenting. He uncomplainingly chauffered the girls to meetings and activities, attended school programs and teachers' conferences and took them on weekend trips that Mommy could not share.

"Hey, I've got something for you, too," I told Ros as I reached into my knitting bag and pulled out a bright blue stocking cap and matching mittens. In the weeks I'd spent at home, I had taught myself to knit, and now family and friends across the United States were sporting my handmade gifts.

"I can't get over you," Ros said. "You've learned to knit, you've sewn each of the girls a new wardrobe, you've redecorated the kitchen and learned to make bread. What next, Wonder Woman?"

I laughed at my friend's new nickname for me. She hurried to the mirror and pulled on her new stocking cap. "Now I'll be all set for our trip to the mountains this weekend."

I sighed. A trip to the mountains sounded like such fun. The only outings I made were to doctors' offices and, aware that there was "something out there that could kill me," I wore a mask over my nose and mouth to protect me from whatever that something was.

The mask didn't live up to its guarantees, however, and four months later my isolation ended abruptly when a tiny germ managed to find its way either through my surgical mask or under my front door to infect me with a respiratory infection that, because of my weak lungs, soon blossomed into a case of double pneumonia complicated with pleurisy.

I was rushed to the hospital on a foggy morning after a night of chest pains, coughing and wheezing. In spite of the unpleasant memories of these sterile institutions, I felt safe and in good hands as a gurney delivered me to the room I was to call home for the next five weeks.

Drifting off to sleep, I looked at the intravenous tube providing nutrition to a vein in my left arm and at the tube through which I was receiving medication in my right. I must look like a machine. Oxygen tubes in my nose and respiratory therapy taken through a hose attached to my mouth surely added to that resemblence.

Thirty-five days is a long time to spend in the hospital, but as I began to feel better, my spirits lifted and I began to make many friends among the therapists, technicians and nurses who cared for me. My room began to look like a greenhouse as friends and family kept me well supplied with roses, carnations and house plants. The once stark walls took on a cheerfulness as they became covered with colorful posters and cards sent by well-wishers.

My sisters, Sally and Jan, were frequent visitors, and they never came empty-handed. Jan kept my room stocked with popcorn and butterscotch candies—my favorite munchies—and Sally always brought along a magazine or book to fill my intellectual appetite. One evening as the intercom announced that visiting hours were over, my sisters decided to hide in the bathroom so that we could continue our conversation. We shut the door and spoke in whispers, but before long we were giggling like naughty children who were afraid to get caught talking after lights out.

Sally had brought me a *Playgirl* magazine that evening, and Jan decided that the handsome, unclad man pictured in the centerfold deserved to be displayed. "Listen, you guys, you can't hang that up in here. It might offend someone." I had to laugh, though, at the thought of stuffy Dr. Adkins confronted by a photo of a nude man on my wall.

"I know. I know." said Jan, with a wicked gleam in her eye. "Let's tack it to the ceiling."

Leave it to Janice. Always mischievous as a child, she hadn't forgotten any of her old tricks. She took off her shoes and stood in the middle of my bed while Sally carefully removed the staples from the full-color centerfold. I rummaged in the drawer for the adhesive tape the nurses kept there and then worked the controls of the bed to raise the mattress as high as possible so that Jan could reach the ceiling.

The deed was accomplished and we all took turns lying on my bed to admire our decorating skills before my sisters kissed me goodnight, tucked me in and sneaked down the hall to the elevator.

The next morning our prank didn't seem so funny, and I was afraid that the medical staff would find my taste objectionable. However, in the remaining two weeks I was there, not one person noticed the adorned ceiling, and I had to hide many a secret smile as the centerfold would catch my eye while I was flat on my back being examined by a round of dignified doctors.

I decided to take advantage of the long, quiet afternoons by reading everything I could find on the subject of allergy. What better place than a hospital environment to do such research, I reasoned. When I had questions, I'd just find a nurse or intern willing to define a term or explain a process I didn't understand. Right?

Wrong.

Most of the medical profession I encountered preferred to speak in vague generalities to their patients. The old cliche "What you don't know won't hurt you" seemed to be their philosophy.

"Don't worry your pretty little head about that. Your doctor will take care of you."

"You just concentrate on getting well, and leave the research to us."

Nonetheless, I struggled through the texts and managed to get a somewhat better understanding of the malfunctioning of my body.

Propped up in bed, with books surrounding me, I found that allergy was, by far, the leading cause of the wheezing, rattling and shortness of breath that asthmatics suffer—and that the hypersensitivity begins with the faulty performance of the body's immune system.

Everyone has inborn defenses that protect them from germs, deadly viruses, bacteria, parasites and other harmful invaders, I read. People have protective mechanisms to fight these dangerous substances and to safeguard their bodies from disease. For instance, everyone, not just asthmatics, has reactive airways that will close down if provoked by noxious fumes. I could remember reading newspaper accounts of trains derailing and spilling some poisonous gas or another, causing the evacuation of whole towns. That made sense, since everyone has built-in reflexes that close airways to protect their bodies from dangerous gases.

In the case of allergic asthma, I found, the immune system begins to work overtime and attempts to do battle with even common elements of everyday life. Along with attacking germs and viruses, some bodies go to war against cat hair, ragweed, house dust, certain foods or a host of other innocuous substances.

What was my body attacking? What kind of a battle was it waging? Would I ever find out? It seemed that answering one question merely led to a dozen others.

I put my large stack of books aside and closed my eyes. Except for the ache I felt from missing my daughters so much, I was feeling better than I had in years. Perhaps the rest and recuperation were just what I needed, but I nonetheless anxiously awaited the doctor's release, promised for the upcoming weekend.

My hopes were dashed, however, when the next day I suffered another anaphylactic attack after eating a meal that was sent up from the hospital kitchen. Though a code-blue alert sent emergency help to my room to revive me almost immediately, nothing could revive my spirits. I fell into a deep depression, requesting that the shades in my room be pulled, that a "Do Not Disturb" sign be posted on my door and that no phone calls be put through to my bed. I told my doctor that I wanted no more tests, no more needles, no more poking and prodding. I just wanted to die in peace.

Dr. Adkins had other plans, however, and wanted to call in a prominent pulmonary specialist.

"No."

"Carolyn, Dr. Paisley is very highly regarded in his field."

"No."

"I've already discussed your case with him and he's said that he thinks he can help you."

Despite my protestations, a spark of hope began to be rekindled within me as Dr. Adkins continued to expound on the specialist's credentials. I agreed to subject myself to yet another series of tests ordered by Dr. Paisley.

The next morning I was given a pill to relax me and was taken to the x-ray department deep in the facility's basement. The bronchogram I was to undergo was considered minor surgery but soon after being wheeled into the small, drab room, I began to wish that the procedure was to be done under general anesthesia instead.

"Stand up right here, Carolyn," one of the two technicians said, arranging my limbs and head in strange positions to accommodate the upcoming test.

"Now, we're going to tie your hands loosely behind your back so your motor reflexes won't cause you to pull out the tube we're going to insert, okay?"

Despite the effects of the tranquilizer, I began to feel anxious about what would happen next. While one technician held my head, the other began to insert a long, rubber tube down my nose. My eyes widened with fear and pain as he continued to push it into my trachea, and through my mind flashed an image of a shackled doe I had seen recently on a television wildlife program.

"Uhh. Uhh." I tried to ask him to stop, but the tubing invading my throat made it impossible for me to communicate. Finally the technician stopped. I wanted to close my eyes and my mind to what was happening, but something compelled me to continue watching.

Approximately a foot of the thin, white tube still stuck out of my right nostril and I was mesmerized as it began to sway up and down and back and forth. The man in the green surgical overblouse turned and reached for what looked like a tube of toothpaste on the counter beside him. As the technician behind me tightened his grip on my head, the first man screwed the "toothpaste" onto the tubing extending from my nose and began to squeeze its contents into my lungs.

"I'm injecting a dye to illuminate your respiratory tract now," the technician explained in a voice one would use to address a child. "Then we'll take a pretty picture of your lungs."

Once the ordeal was over, I returned to my room where my parents were waiting for me. Jerry, unable to cope with my continued illness and the responsibility of the children, had left the girls with neighbors and was off enjoying a week-long fishing trip with friends. At the moment, however, I preferred the role of child more than that of wife, and I welcomed the warm and loving arms of my mother.

"Hold me, Mommy. Just hold me."

I *never* wanted to go through that again.

But I did. Three more bronchograms were required before Dr. Paisley got the "pretty pictures" he required.

Completely exhausted from the week's experience, I was resting against my pillow with my head turned toward the wall when Dr. Paisley hurried into my room late one afternoon.

"Come with me. I have something to show you." He urged me to put on my robe and took my arm almost conspiratorily as he led me to a conference room on the next wing. Entering the long, empty room, my attention was caught by the x-rays backlighted on the opposite wall.

"These are your lungs, Carolyn. See how the dye makes it possible for us to view what normal x-rays can't show?"

Fascinated by the films, I listened as Dr. Paisley explained my problem.

"Lungs look a lot like upside down trees," the physician said, pointing out the similarities of the trachea to a tree trunk, the bronchial tubes to branches and the air sacs to leaves.

"See how nice and wide the 'tree branches' are in your right lung," he asked, his hand sweeping over the area he was describing. "But here in your left lung, the lower branch is shut off. The dye could not enter the tiny twigs, or bronchiole.

"You have a disease called bronchiectasis," he said and explained that the "tree branches" in the lower lobe of my left lung were dead. Bacteria pooled there, providing a perfect breeding ground for my continual infections.

"Your asthma is most assuredly caused by those infections, not by allergy," he told me. "By removing the diseased area, we can correct your problem. Not only will it cure your asthma, but you'll be able to return to a normally active life."

Grasping the specialist's hand, I held it to my cheek to convey my thanks. I was so overcome with tears of gratitude that I could not speak.

Later, unable to sleep, an uneasy thought kept nagging me. Wasn't removal of a lung a terribly drastic step to take to cure asthma? And the left lung, too. Wasn't that dangerously close to the heart? And what bearing did bronchiectasis have on the anaphylactic reactions that had supposedly caused my three life-threatening episodes?

Well, I had three months to get used to the idea of surgery. Dr. Paisley was participating in a boat regatta and wouldn't be able to perform the operation until October. I pushed the doubts and fears from my mind and made myself concentrate on how wonderful it would be to be well again.

Out, damn spot, I quoted to myself, smiling in the dark. If thy left lung offends thee, pluck it out.

Take the lower lobe of my lung, I felt like shouting.

Take the whole damn thing.

Just let me get back to the business of living.

5

"If I should die before I wake, I pray the Lord my soul to take."

Two pair of little hands clasped together tightly. Two pair of eyes squeezed shut. Two tiny voices chimed the sing-song prayer.

"Amen."

Kathy and Meri's big brown eyes flew open and four chubby arms reached out for goodnight hugs and kisses.

"Don't let the bed bugs bite," I said, reaching under the covers to pinch and tweak my older daughter's bottom. Leaving her squealing and laughing, I turned to the other side of the room to repeat the nightly ritual there.

"Goodnight, girls. See you in the morning."

I closed the door of the room Kathy and Meri shared and walked across the hall to my own bedroom.

If I should die before I wake . . . If I should die before I wake. The words of the children's prayer taunted me.

Since arriving home from the hospital a month before, my mind had often been troubled by my upcoming surgery and by the fear of death. Some of my friends worried that I was obsessed with the thought, but it was a feeling I could not seem to shake.

I had been honest about my apprehensions with Jerry and had several long talks with him, needing to know how he would raise the children without me. I made him vow to marry again so my babies would have a mother, made him swear to take them to the doctor when they were sick, made him promise to stay in close touch with my parents, whom the girls adored.

I spent hours copying favorite recipes from cookbooks, and from memory, so that, as a widower, Jerry would be able to prepare fast, nutritious meals for himself and the girls. To further ease my mind, I made arrangements for my body to be cremated when I died and wrote the Forest Service for permission to have my ashes scattered from the mountains near my home. I compiled a long list of friends phone numbers and gave them to my sister, Jan, asking her to call people if I died, to protect Jerry from the unpleasant task.

And, finally, I planned my own memorial service. I detested funerals, found them macabre and grim affairs. I made my friends promise to get together for an hour or two, with Neil Diamond singing "Sweet Caroline" and "Done Too Soon" in the background, to talk and laugh—and cry—about all the good times we'd had together.

Now, with all of those details worked out to my satisfaction, I felt I was more ready to meet the surgeon—and my maker, if necessary.

Instead, I met Mrs. Dunn.

"Are we almost there, Mommy? Are we almost there?"

"Kathy, don't be so impatient! We're about five minutes closer than we were the last time you asked."

In spite of my exasperation, I had to smile. The girls were so excited. We were on our way to Palm Springs—and a mini-vacation before school started the next week. Jerry couldn't afford to take any more time off, but we had talked it over and decided that it was important for the girls to do something special. They had experienced a traumatic summer, staying with one relative and friend after another while they wondered if their mother would ever come home from the hospital. Three days to swim and soak up the sun—and to have their mother's undivided attention—would be the perfect way to end the summer. Besides, I loved Palm Springs. The hot, dry climate had better results on my asthma than any medication I could take, and I knew the desert sun would relax me and take my mind off the surgery I faced.

"There's the turn-off, girls. Look. Palm Springs, 10 miles."

"Hooray. Hooray." Jumping up and down as much as their seat belts would allow, Kathy and Meri talked excitedly of shopping for new bathing suits, staying in a "real live" hotel and eating in restaurants "just like on TV." Poor kids, they hadn't done much traveling. And, on our budget, the "real live" hotel would have to be a Motel 6—and dining out meant one of the fast-food restaurants in town.

We checked into our stark but adequate room, dropped off our suitcases and spent the rest of the morning bargain hunting for bathing suits in the little shops on Palm Canyon Drive. The streets were almost deserted. Who else was crazy enough to even visit Palm Springs in early September, let alone go shopping in 125-degree heat? As the girls began to wilt, however, I realized that the sun's rays weren't a balm to everyone, so we hurriedly decided on matching suits for the two of them, a halter and shorts for me, and jumped back in the car to head for the cool water of the motel's swimming pool.

I noticed the strange little woman the minute we entered the grassy area surrounding the pool. My God, that person looks like a skeleton, I thought. She can't weigh more than 90 pounds.

"Can we go in the water now, Mommy? Can we? Can we?"

"Okay, kids, jump in. But remember all the rules we talked about on our way here."

Off and running, Kathy and Meri headed for the shallow end of the pool, and I was glad once again for the olive complexions that would protect them from the lobster-red sunburn I'd probably have by that evening. I found a chaise longue and sank into its comfortable curve.

And, though I kept one eye on the two bobbing heads in the pool, my attention kept being distracted by the tiny woman sitting in a matching chaise longue to my right. Though the sun was high and the temperature sizzling, she wore a heavy sweater and a little knitted cap. Her eyes were closed, and her arms were crossed over her chest as if even the Palm Springs climate wasn't enough to warm her.

She must be very ill, I thought, and was once again thankful that *my* disease, at least, didn't show from the outside.

The day passed quickly and it was soon time to take the girls in for showers before dressing for dinner and walking to the motel's coffee shop. After a day of sunshine and swimming, both daughters were exhausted and, with tummies filled with hamburgers and malts, they were quite content to be led back to the room and to be tucked into bed for the night.

The next morning we headed back to the coffee shop for breakfast and, as we waited to be seated, the woman I'd noticed the day before walked in the door behind us. I had seen her last night at dinner, also. She had been eating alone, her scrawny body dwarfed by the brown vinyl padding of the restaurant booth.

We smiled at each other, and knowing she must have recognized me and the girls as motel "neighbors," I asked her if she'd like to sit with us at breakfast.

"Why, thank you, dear. I'd love to. Mealtimes can be so lonely."

We moved toward our table, the girls skipping ahead and the older woman more or less shuffling behind. We slipped into a window booth and all introduced ourselves. Her name was Mrs. Dunn, and something about her reminded me of my grandmother. She began talking to the children to overcome their shyness, asking them about school and their pets, so I had a chance to scrutinize our breakfast companion.

She was probably five feet six or seven inches, almost as tall as I, but her extreme thinness made her look like a refugee from the concentration camps I had seen in old World War II newsreels. Despite the heat, she wore long pants and a turtleneck sweater. Her clothes hung on her emaciated frame, and the wedding band she wore was circled with adhesive tape on the back to make it fit. She hadn't always been so skinny.

"Will you be staying in Palm Springs long?" she asked, turning her attention to me.

"No, we're just spending a couple of days here before the girls start school next week. And you?"

I thought the question was appropriate. But I was afraid I sounded more curious than polite.

"Oh, I've been here several weeks already and it looks as if I'll be here several more," said Mrs. Dunn. Her smile pulled the transluscent skin of her face even more tightly across her cheeks. "It's lonely during the weekdays, but my husband and son come out from Los Angeles to spend the weekends with me."

"That's nice. How many children do you have?" I asked, trying to make conversation.

"Just Bobby. He's twelve."

I was surprised to find she had a child so young. I had originally guess her age at 60, but now, after having observed her more closely and after hearing her talk, I doubted she was more than 45.

"Well, I love to spend occasional weeks in Palm Springs, but I don't think I'd like to spend months here—especially alone," I said, sympathizing with her situation.

The waitress brought our breakfasts—chocolate milk and large stacks of pecan pancakes dripping with caramel topping for the girls and a more traditional meal of eggs and bacon for Mrs. Dunn and me.

I had to laugh as Kathy and Meri dove into their hot cakes. "That looks more like dessert than breakfast to me," I teased them. They just smiled and kept eating.

I turned to Mrs. Dunn once again and, unable to contain my inquisitiveness any longer, asked, "Are you here for your health?"

"Yes. The doctor thinks the warm climate and clear air will speed the recuperation process."

Poor thing. I bet she has a terminal illness, I thought. Maybe *my* condition wasn't so bad after all. After meeting Mrs. Dunn I realized things could be worse.

Kathy, who had been listening to the entire conversation, spoke with the bluntness of childhood curiosity. "What's wrong with you?"

"Kathy, it's not polite to ask such personal questions," I scolded my daughter, although I had been dying to ask that very question myself.

"That's all right, dear. I don't mind. I underwent surgery three months ago," she said to Kathy. "The doctor had to take out one of my lungs."

I don't know how I got out of that restaurant. One minute the walls were closing in on me and my breakfast was rushing up into my throat and the next minute I was out in the early morning sunshine, rushing toward my room and yanking the girls along behind me.

"What's wrong, Mommy? Why couldn't we finish our breakfast?" asked Kathy. "Are you mad at that nice lady?"

Instead of answering, I quickened my pace. I was feeling short of breath, but this time it was from panic, not asthma. I felt as if I'd seen a ghost. A ghost of the future. A premonition of what the years ahead held for me.

I had to get away from this motel.

I had to get away from Palm Springs.

And most of all, I had to get away from Mrs. Dunn.

Looking at her was like looking into a crystal ball, and I couldn't cope with what I saw.

6

A second opinion. That's what I needed. After all, that was the rational, astute course to follow for any patient facing a major medical procedure. I tried to ignore the fact that I'd already received five "second opinions" since my asthma had been diagnosed.

I'd find someone new to help me. Someone I could trust. Someone who would listen. Someone who was willing to do something other than overmedicate me or chop out one of my lungs as a solution. But where to find that someone? Where to start looking?

It was 9 a.m. Jerry had been off to work for two hours, and I had just kissed the girls goodbye and sent them on their way to school. Another long, lonely day stretched ahead.

I walked into the kitchen and over to the radio, turning the dial to my favorite station.

"Good morning. This is the Bill Michaels Show. Welcome to KTAK, your talk radio station for Southern California."

Thank heavens for Bill Michaels. He kept me company every morning with a wide variety of interesting guests. Since dropping out of school, I found talk radio a stimulating way to keep abreast of current events, to explore controversial issues and, most of all, to fill the lonesome hours as I went about my chores.

I walked to the pantry, grabbed the flour and shortening and put some milk on the stove to scald. Soon the smell of baking bread would permeate the house.

"My guest this hour is a woman who claims she has the power to heal. The gift of curing the ill. The ability to lay on hands and to restore health to the diseased," said Michaels in his strong, deep broadcaster's voice. "Sister Lucinda Dawn is a psychic healer, and if *you'd* like to talk with her today, here are the numbers you should call."

I stirred a packet of yeast into a cup of warm water. This should be interesting, I thought, and smirked when Michaels described how the switchboard was lighting up as the desperate began inundating the station with calls for miracles from this omnipotent lady.

"Sister. It's so wonderful to talk with you," said the first caller. "My name is Gladys, and I suffer so from migraine headaches. Can you help me?"

As if her powers could travel through the telephone lines! Who would believe such garbage? What kind of person would contact a radio studio to beg help of a clairvoyant who could allegedly cure everything from hang nails to paralysis by a mere touch of her hands?

In spite of my cynicism, I found myself mesmerized. Punching and kneading the ball of dough on the bread board, I listened intently as caller after caller spoke to Sister Lucinda, asking her for help or testifying to the spiritualist's powers. I divided the dough, left it on the counter to rise and, without even washing my hands, sat down in front of the radio and stared at the dial.

"Sister, thank you for helping my brother. He regained his sight after attending your meeting in Portland last year . . . ."

"Please, Sister. My baby was born with spina bifida . . . ."

"Bless you, Sister. I have a new life since I met you in Springfield . . . ."

The calls went on and on, and each person who phoned was answered thoughtfully and, yes, lovingly, by Sister Lucinda Dawn. The woman's charisma and warmth were evident even over the radio.

What would it be like to actually meet her?

"Sister Lucinda, thank you for coming by today. Why don't you tell our listeners where you'll be tonight?"

Despite the dough drying and cracking on my fingers, I rummaged through the drawer by the phone until I found a pencil and piece of paper. I couldn't resist the urge to write down the address of the auditorium where Sister would be speaking that evening at eight.

What am I doing? This is crazy. People like Sister Lucinda Dawn are nothing but quacks. Yet, throughout the morning as I baked my bread and cleaned the kitchen, I continued to think about the psychic and the testimonials I'd heard.

When my own sister, Sally, called from her office during her lunch hour, I began telling her about the medium and her professed abilities to cure.

"Would you like to go hear her speak tonight?" Sally asked. "It certainly couldn't do any harm. Besides, it might be an interesting experience. We'll go together."

What a wonderful sister and friend I had. No ridicule. No scorn. Not a hint of disapproval or mockery. Just love and support—and the willingness to accompany me no matter what path I took. We made arrangements to meet at 6 p.m. to make the long drive into L.A. And I smiled all day as I remembered Sally's parting words as we hung up. "Never underestimate the power of a sister."

That evening, after braving the unfamiliar maze of the rush-hour traffic, Sally and I arrived at the large auditorium with only minutes to spare. A banner, proclaiming "Welcome, Sister" hung over the entrance and a long line of people snaked around the building as the faithful waited to purchase their admittance tickets. I was nervous as we purchased a program and joined the milling crowd attempting to find seats in the rapidly filling audience. Though I considered myself an agnostic, the organ music playing in the background and the churchly atmosphere evoked a strong emotion in me, and I realized that I had not completely abandoned my religious upbringing. I felt the tears rush to my eyes.

"Please, God. I don't know where to turn anymore. Please help me."

A large chorus was first on the agenda, and the lively men and women danced around the stage singing "I Believe in Miracles," generating a frenzied, emotional response from those who had flocked to the auditorium for a combination of spiritualism and the supernatural. The singers invited audience participation, and Sally and I began singing along to some of our favorite old hymns, harmonizing to "Jesus, Jesus, Jesus" and "Standing on the Promises." When the chorus left the stage, the lights dimmed and a drum roll began slowly, soon rising in intensity. The audience began to clap hands and stomp feet in time to the beat.

"Sis-ter. Sis-ter. Sis-ter. Sis-ter." A chant began in the balcony and grew to a crescendo as those on the lower floor joined in the incantation. Sally and I looked at each other, wondering what was coming next.

"I think we're in the midst of a cult," she said over the roar of the crowd.

Before I could reply, the drum ceased to pound and a spotlight dramatically began to play on the red velvet backdrop on stage. A hush came over the audience and, to the melodic strains of "Have Thine Own Way, Lord," Sister Lucinda Dawn stepped through the curtain.

She was a small, trim woman and wore a long, flowing gown of emerald green. Her auburn hair was piled in a mass of ringlets on top of her head, and I guessed her age to be about 45. Holding out her arms as if to embrace us all, Sister Lucinda began to dramatically recite the hymn playing in the background. "Have thine own way, Lord. Have thine own way. Thou art the potter. I am the clay."

She explained in a soothing voice that any healing that might flow from her hands that evening and any cures that might result from her ministrations would actually be the work of God.

The program passed in a rush of prayers, songs, prayers, testimonials, prayers and more prayers—all to the spirited chorus of "Praise the Lord" and "Hallelujah" from the audience. At one point, Sister Lucinda stepped into the aisles, moving swiftly from row to row as people reached out to touch her, to bless her, to hand her pieces of paper bearing the names of those who would like her to intercede on their behalf with the man on high.

Next on the program was an offering. Donations were solicited so that Sister could continue her good work, we were told. Spreading the Lord's word was apparently an expensive endeavor. I was surprised to see people reaching into their pockets, opening their purses, slipping bills out of their wallets and generously filling the offering trays as they slowly made their way up and down each row of the large assembly hall.

"My God, people have already paid five dollars each to get in here," I whispered to Sally. My eyes widened as the large silver tray was passed to me and I noted the overflowing collection of bills—fives, tens and even twenties.

After the offering was ushered onto the stage and taken quickly out of sight behind the curtain, I felt myself caught up once again by the soft, familiar music of my Sunday School days and the mellow, almost hypnotic voice of Sister Lucinda inviting the tired, the sick, the aged and the diseased to join her on stage for the moment we'd all been waiting for—the laying on of hands, the healing for which we had all gathered.

Sally and I exchanged a long look, and I felt myself torn by conflicting thoughts. I had renounced my church—and my God—years before. I had rejected the teachings of the Bible and left behind the religion that had been so much a part of my youth. Wasn't I a hypocrite to be here now? Wouldn't God—and Sister Lucinda Dawn—realize that I had no right to ask for divine intervention after forsaking my faith for all these years? Yet, like a despairing soldier offering up a foxhole prayer, I wanted so much to believe.

What if this woman really could cure me? I'd heard the claims. I'd seen the people who testified that they'd been crippled before Sister's hands had performed their magic. If I had enough trust would my lungs turn pink and healthy and unrestricted?

Sally's eyes filled with tears, and she hugged me close. "Go on down, Carolyn. What do you have to lose?"

I took a deep breath, stood up and climbed over the people in my row until I finally reached the aisle and joined those wending their ways to the large stage. Twisted spastic children were carried forward by their mothers and fathers. Enfeebled senior citizens with shawls and blankets covering shriveled legs and limbs were pushed ahead in wheelchairs. People with braces lurched toward the open arms Sister Lucinda was extending. Men and women on crutches swung their crippled bodies in the direction of a hoped-for miracle.

Moving forward with this desperate flow of humanity, I knew I looked out of place. My disease lay within me and was disguised by my young and deceivingly healthy-looking body.

It took more than an hour for us all to file by Sister Lucinda Dawn. She sat in a large velvet chair in the center of the stage—almost as if she were a queen holding court. As each person paused in front of her, she reached toward the afflicted part of the body, running her hands gently over frail legs, contorted backs, knotted arthritic hands and bent gray heads, offering a prayer and a private word with each hopeful soul.

When it was my turn to stand before the psychic, she stood up so that she could gaze into my eyes. She clasped both of my arms tightly and closed her eyes, her lips moving in silent prayer. When she was finished, her eyes once again held mine and she moved her hands softly in front of me, encompassing my body from head to foot.

"The doctor is on the right track," she told me serenely, then turned her attention immediately to the little old woman in the wheelchair behind me.

Tears blinded me, but I somehow managed to get down the stairs without falling. Sally was waiting at the foot of the stage, and I almost collapsed as I rushed into her arms and wept. Recognizing my emotion as one of desolation rather than the joy we had hoped for, she led me out a side door and back to the privacy of the car. We sat there for 20 minutes, Sally attempting to console me as I mourned yet another closed door in my search for a cure.

"She said the doctor was on the right track," I finally was able to tell her. "I think Sister Lucinda and God are in cahoots with Dr. Paisley."

I tried to make light of the situation, but I felt the grief welling up inside me and tears once again began to flow.

We made the long drive back to Orange County in total silence.

I glanced down at the program I still clutched in my fist and at Sister Lucinda's benign face peering up at me from the cover. I crumpled the brochure in my hands, wrinkling the paper and turning the spiritualist's smile into a twisted and almost mocking leer.

Now what, I wondered hopelessly. I'd tried a shrink. I'd been to the "best" doctors. A faith healer hadn't been the answer.

Wasn't there anyone who could help?

7

W*alk briskly for ten breaths, walk slowly for ten breaths. Walk briskly for ten breaths, walk slowly for ten breaths.*

Placing one foot in front of the other and swinging my arms as I walked the perimeter around my housing tract, I counted off the inhalations and matched my steps to the rhythm of my silent chant.

After the fiasco with Sister Lucinda Dawn, I'd felt depressed about my condition and my inability to steer the course of my own life. Yet still I couldn't accept the fact that surgery was my only hope. I once again began to frequent both the college and public libraries in my area, hoping to find another, less drastic route to better health.

Exercise was one of the programs I'd decided to follow. Would it help? I wasn't sure. But at least it wouldn't hurt—and it was certainly worth a try. I'd just read that five medal winners in the 1972 Olympics were asthmatics. Not that I wanted to ever compete or set records, but the knowledge that it *was* possible had certainly impressed me.

I rounded the last corner of my half-mile jaunt and began to slow my pace, conscious of the fact that a "cooling off" period was as important to an asthmatic as was a "warm up" time. I consciously kept my arms from swinging and slowed my steps even more to reduce the "oxygen-debt" that people usually experience at the end of their exercise period.

I couldn't believe I was doing this. I'd always hated exercising and had never enjoyed the physical education classes I'd been required to take in high school. In fact, in recent years, I was quick to use my asthma as an excuse to avoid *any* kind of exertion. It surprised me to discover, then, that asthmatics could receive real benefits from aerobic types of exercise—the kind that made the heart beat fast, the lungs expand and the blood vessels open wide to carry oxygen-enriched blood to the cells.

I laughed to myself as I remembered the book I'd read by Dr. Henry Hyde Salter, *On Asthma*, written in 1864. "Organs are made for action, not existence," he wrote more than a century ago. "They are made to *work*, not to *be;* and when they work well, they can be well."

Okay, Dr. Salter. I'll give it a whirl. If nothing else, my daily walks were putting color back in my cheeks and were getting me out of the house for awhile each morning. I could see my little white stucco house up ahead of me now and resisted the urge to quicken my pace.

Maybe I'd finally learn to swim. Swimming, I'd read, was the best exercise for asthmatics. It had something to do with the warm, humid air that hovers over a pool area. The tissues of the lungs didn't lose moisture in such an environment. Swimming also strengthened the chest muscles, I'd learned. I grinned as I sauntered along. Maybe I could build up my bust and improve my lung capacity at the same time. The best thing about swimming though, according to my research, was that the controlled breathing necessary to keep from drowning—and breathing out against the pressure of the water—caused a more efficient exchange of air. All I had to do was overcome my fear of water and find a place that offered adult lessons.

I climbed the steps to my front door and let myself into my small but comfortable home. I promptly dispensed a glass of the bottled water we'd begun to have delivered weekly. To my myriad medications, I had added at least 10 tall glasses of water each day. I actually sloshed when I walked, but I'd read that water could reduce the stickiness of sputum and could keep mucus loose so that it could be coughed up and kept from blocking the bronchial tubes. I wondered why none of my doctors had told me that water is the best expectorant.

Doctors had never mentioned the value of vitamins either, and though I knew there were no guarantees as to the results, I now took vitamins A, C, and E. Vitamin A is important in maintaining the cells that line the respiratory tract, I had read. Vitamin E reportedly protects lung cells from exposure to air pollution and Vitamin C is said to decrease a person's chances of catching colds—which always meant lung infections, bronchitis or even pneumonia for me.

The phone rang, and I drained my glass of the last ounce of water and rushed over to pick up the receiver.

"Hello?"

My mother's concerned voice answered. "Honey, are you all right? I've been calling for over an hour. I've been worried to death."

I sighed. "I'm fine, Mom. I was just out taking a walk."

My poor family. It seemed that everyone suffered as much from my asthma as I did. They also lived in fear of my next attack.

Relieved that I had not turned blue somewhere or been rushed once again to a hospital, my mother relaxed and told me why she had called.

"Honey, when I was reading the newspaper this morning I saw an advertisement that discussed a new process for controlling asthma and other allergies. It involves injecting the patient with his own . . ." She lowered her voice to a whisper. ". . . Well, his own urine."

"What?"

I had to laugh, and Mom laughed right along with me. It did sound rather unusual—and certainly unorthodox.

"That's the strangest cure I've ever heard, Mom. How in the world would urine affect asthma?"

"Well, to tell you the truth, I really didn't understand it," my mother admitted, "but I clipped it out and sent it along with the postman. You'll probably receive it in the mail tomorrow."

And I did. I eagerly awaited the mailman the next day and ran out to the curb to greet him as he drove his little cart to the end of my driveway. There it was—a letter addressed in my mother's large, loopy handwriting.

I tore the envelope open as I returned to the house. God, I must be grasping at straws if I were so anxious to read about cures brought about by urine injections. It sounded so disgusting. But not half as disgusting as having a lung removed, a little voice inside my head reminded me.

Sitting down on the couch, I glanced at the large quarter-page ad. It attempted to simulate a newspaper article, complete with headline and a photo of a smiling patient receiving a shot from a dark-haired young doctor. "New Allergy Treatment Considered a Medical Breakthrough" the bold type declared. Only the word "advertisement" in small capital letters at the bottom of the boxed-in copy told readers it was not a news story concerning a scientific discovery.

My suspicions were aroused immediately. If this procedure were as revolutionary and foolproof as the claims said, why *wasn't* there a bona fide article written by a medical editor instead of a paid announcement? On the other hand, the medical community wasn't always willing to accept new methods of treatment without years and years of study and testing. And I didn't have years and years to waste.

I began to read, my eyes flying over the newsprint. Maybe this whole thing wasn't so bizarre after all. According to the theory, people who were allergic breathed in or ingested substances to which they reacted with sniffles, watery eyes, wheezes and the like. These substances ended up in the bladder and formed a balanced allergen solution. Desensitizing the body with injections of a fluid containing the very cause of the allergy, rather than injecting it with an approximate serum from a laboratory somewhere was extremely beneficial to the allergy-sufferer and much more effective than current methods, I read.

That made sense. It really did. I had no idea what was causing my asthma, but if it were an allergy, this treatment might help. The culprit, that unknown "something" I was allergic to, would end up in my urine. By receiving injections that contained that "something," my body could build up an immunity to it and my problem would be solved.

I anxiously awaited Jerry's return home that night. He had taken scores of science courses in high school and college, and his years as a chemist made him much better educated than I about subjects such as this.

I hurried through dinner, sent the girls off to play and sat down once again at the dining room table where my husband was finishing his last cup of coffee. Excitedly I told him of the new theory. He didn't sound as convinced as I about its merits, however, and he wasn't certain about the conclusions I'd drawn concerning my own case.

"I don't know, Babe. There's something strange about this. Why don't you ask one of your doctors about it before you decide to make an appointment."

But who to ask? Dr. Adkins had brought Dr. Paisley in on my case and agreed wholeheartedly with the diagnosis of bronchiectasis. Dr. Whitmore had tried desensitizing me to no avail, and he had never been anxious to discuss my theories with me in the past. I was afraid he'd react just as unkindly to any conversation in which I'd offer suggestions now.

What gave doctors such God complexes anyway? Why did they think that only they had all the answers? I was becoming quite cynical and disillusioned with the medical profession. The only doctor left who I felt I could trust was my gynecologist.

I sat up straight in my chair. Why not? Why not ask my Ob/Gyn for advice. He wasn't involved with the care of my asthma. Perhaps his opinion would be unbiased on this subject. It was worth a phone call to find out.

Dr. Rice returned my call the next day. Since the birth of my children, I'd only seen him once a year for my annual pap smear. Nonetheless, he still remembered me and his voice was as warm and caring as ever.

"Carolyn, it's been quite a while since we've seen you. Isn't it about time for you to drop by for a visit?"

"I'll make an appointment to see you in a couple of months, doctor. But I've called you for advice on a different subject today."

I once again expounded the urine-injection theory, making sure to relate its benefits to my own disease.

There was silence on the other end of the line and for a moment I thought we'd been disconnected. Then I heard him clear his throat.

"Hocus-pocus," he said in a grave voice, devoid of its usual friendliness.

"Pardon me?"

"Carolyn, this procedure is nothing but a scam, believe me. I know you're anxious to find something to help you but, honestly dear, this so-called new treatment is not what you're looking for."

I put the receiver to my other ear and continued to listen to my doctor's cool, yet determined tirade.

"First of all, the quantity of allergen in the urine would be an infinitestimal part of what you'd need to become immune. The entire theory has no foundation in reality. These laboratories, and I use the term loosely, are nothing but money-making machines for unscrupulous doctors who move from city to city taking advantage of unsuspecting and desperate patients."

"Like me," I said in a small, tired voice, finishing his sentence for him.

Dr. Rice's voice returned to its well-modulated pitch and once again carried the warmth I had come to expect from him.

"Think about it, dear. Does it make sense to urinate into a jar and then pay someone hundreds of dollars to inject your body's waste back into your tissues?"

No, I guess it didn't make sense after all. I thanked Dr. Rice for returning my call and for his candid opinion before saying goodbye and hanging up. I remained sitting there, staring at the phone.

Where could I turn next?

The next week, Jerry came home with a note sent by friends from work.

> *Dear Carolyn,*
> *We're so sorry to hear about your continued problems. Have you considered making an appointment at Scripps Clinic and Research Foundation? The place has a wonderful reputation, and we have another friend who was really helped by going there. Stay well. We hope to see you both soon.*
>
> *—Dick and Peg*

I'd heard of Scripps, of course. It was just 100 miles south of us in the seaside community of La Jolla. But they only accepted patients with rare conditions—or so I thought. Would they be willing to see me?

Yes, they assured me when I called the next day. One of the doctors in their allergy department would be glad to discuss my case. However, it would help if I had my records and a letter of recommendation sent to them from my allergist in Long Beach.

I made an appointment with Dr. Whitmore immediately, and when he discovered I was there, not for an examination, but to pick up my records, he reacted as if I'd insulted him.

"I'll give you a referral letter if that's what you want," he said, his eyes boring into mine. "But they'll just tell you the same thing I have—and charge you two or three thousand dollars to do so."

I returned Dr. Whitmore's icy stare. I had visited his office more times than I could count. I'd been a faithful patient, obediently taking his orders, his injections, his advice for years. I'd spent thousands upon thousands of dollars to hear his final recommendation that I never leave my home if I wanted to see my children grow up. If anyone were in the position to be taking offense, it should be me.

Gathering every ounce of dignity I could, I stood up and faced Dr. Whitmore. "I'd like that letter and a copy of my records sent to me by Monday. I plan to make an appointment at Scripps as soon as possible."

I turned, opened the door and walked out of the examination room. I never saw Dr. Whitmore again.

8

I don't know what I expected, but the small gray building on a quiet little street in La Jolla certainly didn't fit my image of a world-famous research clinic. The parking lot was cramped and inadequate, and Jerry and I had to circle the streets for blocks before finding a place to leave our car. We walked through the arched doorway and registered with the receptionist, who gave me a handful of papers to fill out. At least they'd keep me busy while we waited.

Forms. Forms. Forms. How many hundreds of them had I filled out in the past few years? Age, sex, height, weight, who to contact in case of emergency, insurance carrier. I could fill these things out with my eyes closed. But, as I worked through the tall stack of papers, I realized these were more thorough than any I'd ever been asked to answer. The questions were in-depth, comprehensive and dealt with times and events dating back to my childhood. There were many I couldn't answer. I'd have to ask my mother for some of the information they wanted.

Within a half hour, a swarthy young man in a white coat walked into the lobby and approached me.

"I'm Dr. Adrian," he said with an accent I couldn't place. "Won't you come back to my office?"

Surprised and impressed, I followed him down the hall and into a small cubicle overlooking the Pacific Ocean. I'd never had a doctor greet me in the waiting room before. It certainly added a personal touch, and one I liked.

However, I wouldn't let myself be taken in by manners. Never again would a doctor automatically receive my trust. Never again would a smile and a concerned attitude be enough to earn my faith. Dr. Adkins had been kind and caring and had turned me into a drugged zombie. Dr. Whitmore had seemed self-assured and competent, and he'd suggested I imprison myself in my home for the rest of my life. Dr. Paisley had been lovable and almost grandfatherly in his care of me—and he'd wanted to mutilate my body and turn me into an invalid like Mrs. Dunn. And the others—the doctor who said I probably wouldn't live to see 40, the doctor who had told me that things could be worse—that I could have cystic fibrosis.

No. This time a nice bedside manner wouldn't suffice. I sat stiffly in

Dr. Adrian's office, my tension mounting and the chip on my shoulder growing by the minute.

Dr. Adrian explained to me that he was from South Africa and worked at the Clinic as a fellow, a graduate student who had been given a grant for further study. Medical allergies were of great interest to him, and he and Dr. Stevens, the staff physician, had been assigned to my case.

With these introductions out of the way, I began to tell Dr. Adrian of my medical history. I also told him of my frustrations and my fears. I finished by conveying Dr. Paisley's diagnosis and subsequent decision to remove my lung.

Dr. Adrian began reading over my forms, frequently asking me a question to verify some of the information and making notes in the margins.

I had been sure to emphasize the fact that I had not had asthma until I was 27 years old, yet the doctor pressed the point that I had mentioned occasional wheezes as a child.

"I didn't have asthma as a girl," I insisted. "I only remember wheezing once or twice in my entire childhood—once it was after laughing really hard at something."

The doctor began to take notes again. "So strong emotion could bring about a wheezing episode."

My nerves were on edge, and the doctor's assumption infuriated me. I began shouting.

"My asthma is *not* brought about by emotion. It is *not* psychosomatic."

I picked up my purse and began gathering the x-rays and records I'd brought with me. I started to cry, and my voice quaked. "I'm sorry I've taken up your time. I think it would be better if I left now."

The young doctor rose quickly and walked to my side. Gently, he took the large envelopes from me and asked me to sit down. He sat on the chair next to me and spoke calmly.

"Carolyn, I know what you've been through these past few years. You have every right to be angry and afraid. I didn't mean to imply that your asthma is caused by emotion—that was a poor way to phrase it and I apologize."

He offered me a Kleenex and I dabbed at my eyes and blew my nose.

"I'd like you to stay," Dr. Adrian said. "I'd like to try to help you."

I took another tissue and tried to mop up the mascara running down my face. I raised my head and looked at Dr. Adrian. His kind face shimmered through my teary eyes. I nodded mutely.

I'd come all this way. I might as well stay. If I didn't like what he had to say after his examination, I could always leave and never come back. I'd give it a chance.

"Thank you," I finally managed to say.

The next four hours were spent in what Dr. Adrian termed a preliminary examination. Preliminary? The allergy staff's preciseness made quite an impact on me—and this was just the beginning of the testing, I was told. I was ushered from lab to lab and was given a methocoline challenge to document the fact that I had asthma. I was given chest and sinus x-rays, blood tests, pulmonary exams and lung function tests. Despite the numerous procedures I underwent and the full schedule that kept me moving from one technician to another, I didn't once feel I was being herded about. I was treated with respect and courtesy. Every member of the department was friendly and seemed genuinely interested in me and my problem. Again I was favorably impressed. It was so different from my other experiences with the medical profession.

At 3 o'clock that afternoon, I finally met Dr. Stevens, a tall, blond, boyishly-handsome man who greeted me warmly and actually asked permission to examine me.

"I know you've been through a lot of tests today, but I'd like to listen to your chest, too, if I may."

I was still wearing the blue striped hospital gown, so it was certainly no imposition to sit on the examination table and to breathe in and out and cough on command as Dr. Stevens ran his stethoscope over my chest and back, listening to the crackles and wheezes emanating from deep within my lungs.

"Why don't you get dressed and come on in my office now," he said when he'd heard enough. "Dr. Adrian and I would like to talk with you."

Here I am again, I thought as I took a seat in the doctor's office. Waiting for yet another diagnosis, another answer. Feeling that my very life was in the balance, I prayed that these doctors would offer a new course of action.

I wasn't disappointed.

"Carolyn, first of all we want to let you know that we've studied your x-rays and have even had doctors from other departments here at the Clinic take a look at them while you were having your other tests conducted this afternoon."

Dr. Stevens took off his glasses, leaned forward and shook his head. "You do *not* have bronchiectasis. There is no sign of any diseased tissue in your lungs. Why the lower lobe of your left lung did not show up after your bronchograms last summer, I don't know. Perhaps that part of your lung was still blocked from the pneumonia you'd had. Maybe the dye itself caused your bronchial tubes to react and constrict. I can only speculate. Anyway, everyone at Scripps Clinic who has seen your x-rays is in agreement—*you do not have bronchiectasis.*"

I was stunned. I was ecstatic. I felt like jumping up and down with glee. I wanted to throw my arms around both Dr. Stevens and Dr. Adrian and hug them in joy. Instead I bawled.

I cried and sobbed for at least fifteen minutes, using up the entire box of Kleenex Dr. Adrian offered me. I kept trying to compose myself and kept choking out that I was sorry to fall apart like this. The doctors—*my* doctors—continued to pat me on the back, squeeze my hand and tell me again and again that my reaction was perfectly all right. They seemed as happy as I, although their delight at the diagnosis took a different form than mine. They beamed instead of blubbered.

Finally my overworked tear ducts gave out and I dried my swollen eyes and listened intently to Dr. Stevens' words.

"You do have asthma, Carolyn, and asthma can be a very serious disease. But with the right medications and a proper program of care, there's no reason you can't live a normal life."

He emphasized each sentence with a flourish of his hands.

"There's no reason at all that you can't leave your house. There's no reason you can't go back to school. There's no reason you can't do anything you want to do."

Was I dreaming? Had I died and gone to heaven? This man was offering me back my life.

"I can't promise you you'll always feel great. I can't promise you you'll never have an asthma attack. We don't know what's causing the anaphylaxis, but we're going to try to find out. In the meantime, we want you to start *living* again."

Dr. Stevens smiled at me with his crooked grin. "Tell me, my friend, has anyone ever really explained asthma to you?"

I stared at him. What an unexpected question. Hadn't I lived with the condition for years? Asthma meant shortness of breath and wheezing all night long. Asthma meant a frightening sensation of suffocation. It meant debilitation, despair, panic . . . .

I continued to look blankly, first at Dr. Stevens and then at Dr. Adrian, unable to formulate an intelligent answer.

As if reading my mind, the doctor answered for me. "Probably no one could describe the *feelings* associated with the disease better than you," he said, "but *technically*, the name asthma comes from the Greek word that means panting, and although our knowledge of asthma is much more extensive today than it was in ancient Greece, it's still a baffling disease."

He leaned forward in his chair, rested his elbows on his desk and began counting on his fingers for emphasis. "It can be caused by allergies, infections, smoke, air pollution, cold air, a change in climate . . . ."

Suddenly Dr. Stevens swiveled in his chair and jumped up to rummage in the small closet next to his desk. He pulled out a chart illustrating the lungs and placed it on his desk, wedging it between some books so that it would stand up.

"As elementary as it may sound, to understand asthma, it is important to first understand the respiratory system—just how and why we breathe."

He took a pencil and began to point at the various parts of the chart. "The air we inhale enters our nose, moves down our throat into the trachea, or windpipe, and on through the bronchial tree to the outermost branches, the air sacs. From the air sacs, which are called the alveoli, oxygen passes into the blood stream. Here also, carbon dioxide is picked up from the bloodstream and expelled in our exhaled air."

I listened attentively. I vaguely remembered all of this from high school biology, but I had never really correlated the information with the breathing difficulties I'd had as an adult.

"The bronchial tree is lined with moist mucous membranes, and the surface is covered with hairlike structures called cilia," Dr. Stevens continued. "As these hairs wave, they move mucus toward the outside of the body, cleaning the surface of the membranes by sweeping them clean of small particles that might have been inhaled. When we breathe in our chests expand in length and breadth."

To illustrate, he took a deep breath, exaggerating the inhalation to almost comically enlarge his chest as if he'd swallowed a balloon.

Dr. Stevens exhaled noisily. "Mother Nature should be congratulated. The respiratory system is a beautiful one and one we take too much for granted—when it's working right."

I urged him to continue his mini-lecture. "But what happens when things don't go right? How do the lungs function during an asthma attack?"

"You might say that Murphy's law goes into effect," Dr. Stevens said. "The smooth muscles of the air passage constrict and tighten, squeezing and narrowing the airways and causing bronchospasm. The lining of the bronchial tubes swell, much like your skin would if you were bitten by a mosquito.

"Mucus is produced in excessive amounts, which plug the tubes and leave little room for air. The body has to work harder to empty and fill the lungs, and stale air is trapped inside. The wheeze associated with asthma is the sound of air being forced out of the shrunken airways, vibrating on the strands of phlegm."

So that's what went on inside my lungs. I couldn't believe it had never been explained to me before. I couldn't believe I'd never asked. I'd always been so intimidated by doctors who made me feel I was wrong to take up their valuable time asking a lot of questions. Dr. Stevens, however, seemed as comfortable in the role of teacher as he did in that of physician.

My thoughts were interrupted as Dr. Adrian asked me if I'd be willing to come back to the Clinic as an in-patient for a week. There were more tests to be given, challenges to be received, medications to be tried.

"I'll stay right now if you'd like me to," I said impulsively, not stopping to think of all the arrangements I'd need to make before spending yet another week in the hospital.

Dr. Stevens and Dr. Adrian laughed. "Don't be such a glutton for punishment," Dr. Stevens said. "You've been through enough today. Go home now and get some rest. Call tomorrow and we'll set it up for a time that's convenient."

I shook hands with both men, although I felt more like kissing them. "Thank you. Thank you both," I said, finding it hard to convey my intense gratitude with those two inadequate little words.

I floated rather than walked back into the lobby where Jerry had been waiting all this time. My eyes were red and puffy and my cheeks were splotchy from crying. My hair was a fright from pulling my clothes on and off over my head all day to undergo the long series of tests. My make-up was streaked and messy. Nonetheless, the smile on my face told my husband what he wanted to know.

As we left Scripps, I turned and once again looked at the gray structure that I'd seen for the first time only hours before. This morning it had seemed nothing more than an old, drab building in desperate need of renovation. But now it was shining in my eyes like a beacon of hope.

9

I walked slowly across the campus of California State University, clutching my purse to my side. Patting its roundness, I felt for the outline of the adrenalin kit through the thin, brown vinyl. I literally carried my life in this handbag.

Despite my doctor's encouragement, returning to school two years before hadn't been easy. Walking from building to building still took all the effort I could muster, and I was grateful that the college had issued me a medical parking permit so that I could at least avoid the long trek from the nether reaches of the massive parking lot.

Resting on one of the concrete benches bordering the sidewalk, I took a deep breath. Not many people have a second chance at life, and I was determined to make the most of mine. I felt lucky that my doctors at Scripps Clinic were optimistic and interested in seeing me improve my quality of life. In the past, physicians had been content by the mere fact that I continued to exist.

I remained huddled on the cold, cement bench, gathering my strength and trying to ignore the curious glances of the other students. I wish they wouldn't stare at me. They should be getting used to the spectacle I presented. I knew I didn't fit in. I was older than most of the students hurrying around the Fullerton campus, but that wasn't the problem. I still looked young enough and, if I'd been wearing recycled faded Levis and a rumpled Madras shirt, I would have been unnoticed among all the other coeds. However, I was constantly plagued by colds that could develop into respiratory infections overnight, so I always dressed warmly and came more prepared for snow, rain and the cold of night than any postman I'd ever known. Oh, sure, this might be sunny California, but the winters were wet and miserable, and I wasn't taking any chances.

After my rest, I was breathing easily once again, so I stood up and plodded on toward class. My large rubber, fur-lined boots made scuffing noises as I walked but, if it rained, they would keep my feet dry. I wore long corduroy pants, a heavy sweater, a water-proof poncho and a scarf to protect my ears—even ear infections could spread to my lungs. I knew. I had found out the hard way.

At the Humanities Building, the escalator wasn't working. Thank God the college nurse had suggested giving me a key to the freight elevator.

The escalators were often out of order, and I would never have been able to climb the stairs to my fifth-floor class.

I walked down the side of the building to the small lift and, with gloved hands, searched for the large gold key in the bottom of my purse. Wrestling with my book bag and the umbrella I always carried, I finally managed to turn the key in the lock and stepped inside as the elevator arrived to carry me to American Studies 422—"Progress in the American Society."

Progress. That's what I was finally beginning to make. Let the other students stare. Let them snicker at my strange wardrobe. I was going to graduate this June. Fourteen long, grueling years after I'd enrolled in my first college class, I actually was going to receive my degree.

Now that was progress.

I only wished I could make as much headway when it came to my health. Since learning to inject myself with adrenalin, I felt confident that I could take care of myself when confronted with the frightening episodes of anaphylaxis. But what was causing them? I decided to begin keeping a journal. Perhaps if I chronicled my activities, my medications, my comings and goings, and yes, even my emotions, I might eventually find some link, some clue, some thread of information that would help me solve this mystery . . . .

> May 29, 1976
>
> I did it! I'm a college graduate—with honors yet. I could hear Jerry and the girls cheering in the audience when they called my name—and Sally surprised me with a party when we returned home.
>
> June 18, 1976
>
> I've got a JOB. Someone is actually paying me to work in their communications department to do the thing I love most—write. Not only am I helping to edit the company publications, they want me to write their history. I'm on my way.
>
> August 3, 1976
>
> Oh, God, it happened again last night. After work a group of us stopped by a Mexican restaurant and were enjoying guacamole and tortilla chips and sipping margaritas when it hit me. I managed to excuse myself and got to the ladies room where I gave myself a shot. I can't describe the terror I feel each time this happens. Will I ever discover what causes it?
>
> September 6, 1976
>
> How can everything be going so well with my career and so lousy at home? Jerry and I seem to be living parallel lives—no common interests, no common goals, not even any friends in common.
>
> November 8, 1976
>
> Kathy's birthday. I am now the mother of a teenage daughter.

Where did the years go? Am I really old enough to have a 13-year-old child?

February 20, 1977

I've been sick, but I told everyone at work it was just a cold—they say they can hear me coughing and wheezing in the next office, even though I keep my door closed. I haven't confided in anyone at the company about my asthma or anaphylaxis—I'm afraid I'd lose my job. I just gulp my pills each morning, drive to work, take the elevator to the third floor and sit at my desk all day writing. I told my doctor it's actually an easier routine than going to school was.

May 19, 1977

I *love* my job. I *love* the stimulation of the business world. Researching and writing the history of this exciting company has been a real joy. Just think—I'll be a published author by next month.

August 4, 1977

The girls and I spent Saturday and Sunday at the beach. They decided to teach me how to body surf—even though I never learned how to swim. I wish Jerry wanted to share these fun times with us

September 23, 1977

One of my semi-annual check-ups at Scripps Clinic. More of the same old thing and no new answers. I've tried every medication to come on the market and none has any measurable effect. I've even gone to Mexico and smuggled some across the border that the FDA has not yet approved. Oh, well, I'll keep giving them a try. What else can I do?

November 16, 1977

Just when my confidence was being restored, it happened again. A steak house this time. God, I've tried so hard to find out why it happens. I'm sure it's got to be cooking fumes coming from the kitchen or cigarette smoke of the other patrons. I've decided not to eat in restaurants anymore. I might not be so lucky next time.

January 24, 1978

A new job. A great opportunity to advance in a company that's just opened a communications department. I'll edit the magazine and write another corporate history. Best of all—a $6,000 a year raise!

June 2, 1978

There's so much tension in my marriage. I can't take any more. I think we both know it's over. But I'm so afraid. Can I take care of the girls by myself? What if I get really sick again?

July 7, 1978

Remember me? I'm the one who's always saying that life is not a rehearsal. I can't stay in a marriage just because I might get sick someday.

August 15, 1978

Well, we finally talked about it. Isn't it strange that, when we finally sat down to communicate, it was to work out details of our divorce rather than our marriage? We've told the children. The four of us hugged and cried all day. Jerry and I promise each other that this thing will be handled amiably and that we'll give Kathy and Meri all of the extra love and support that they need right now.

August 16, 1978

Oh, God. Am I doing the right thing?

10

I stepped on the accelerator and moved my sleek little sports car into the stream of traffic. California rush hour had always had an hypnotic influence on me and, as I inched along with the other commuters, I had time to reflect on the events of the past six months. Yes, I had definitely done the right thing by getting a divorce. It was the only thing I could have done. With the trauma of the courtroom behind me, I was finding my new life exciting and challenging.

I switched on my right turn signal and moved slowly into the adjacent lane. I was headed for home.

Home. It had taken a while before the girls and I had felt we belonged in the two-story condominium I'd bought. It certainly wasn't the roomy four-bedroom house we'd left behind. But with some new furniture and a few decorative touches, it was becoming more comfortable.

I patted the dashboard of my recently purchased Mazda RX-7. In a way, it was a symbol of my new life. I wasn't certain where I was going, but getting there was going to be anything but dull. I loved being on my own and was heady with the power of being truly independent for the first time in my life. Even my health seemed somewhat better—at least my asthma was being well-controlled. And, since I'd stopped eating out, I'd had no further episodes of anaphylactic shock.

I looked skyward and, in spite of the smoggy brown horizon, I found myself quoting Robert Browning. God's in his heaven. All's right with the world.

Of course, the fact that there was a new man in my life couldn't help but contribute to my well-being.

"I can't believe this. *My* mother going out—with a man!"

Kathy and I were going through my closet later that evening, rejecting one outfit after another in our search for the perfect clothes to wear on Mom's First Date.

"Now, Momma, don't be late tonight or we won't let you do this again," Meri said.

Both girls had teased me unmercifully about this new turn in my life. I know it made them uncomfortable to see me with another man, and making light of the situation helped alleviate their anxiety. They were close to their father and saw him often, but by now they had given up any fantasies they might have had that we would someday get back together.

They had met my friend Vick and had liked him right away. He had worked with children all of his life and had a lively sense of humor that put the girls immediately at ease. It surprised me that they so quickly picked up his bantering mood by making jokes about the disparity in our heights and builds. I was a slender 5'8" and Vick was a portly 5'5"—although he insisted we refer to him as 4'17" because it made him sound taller. Similarly, he dispelled any qualms about our 17-year age difference by telling Kathy and Meri that he was only 11 on the Celsius scale.

I smiled to myself. His quick wit had been one of the things that had attracted me when we first met also. He had entered my life several years before, while I was a senior in college. To earn my degree, I had to spend 150 hours working in the field of my choice. I had selected to explore a career in communications and applied for an internship in the community relations department at Childrens Hospital of Orange County.

I had arrived at CHOC in my new "interviewee" suit and, as I took the elevator to the basement offices, I hoped that my age and maturity would be a help rather than a hinderance for the position.

"Hello. Come on in. You're certainly prompt." Vick Knight, the director of development, greeted me enthusiastically. I was barely seated when his secretary gave him a handful of phone messages and suggested he might want to take the call now coming in on line three.

"Excuse me a moment," he said to me, then picked up the phone to carry on an animated conversation with a news reporter who had called regarding a 10-K run being held that weekend to benefit Childrens Hospital.

I was grateful for the opportunity to catch my breath before the interview—and happy for a chance to gather my first impressions about the man who had been described to me as the best public relations practitioner and fund raiser in Orange County.

He looked like a cross between Kenny Rogers and Captain Kangaroo, with his round, smiling face and silver-white hair. Yet there was something elfin about him, too. His blue eyes twinkled and his laugh came frequently during his phone conversation. What captured my attention most, however, was the fact that the man could expend so much energy during a mere telephone call. I watched him spin in his upholstered chair, lean forward to doodle on a pad of paper and then lean back so far in laughter that I was afraid the entire chair would tip over.

He was a human dynamo. I'd have to find out who made his office furniture. If it could take this abuse, I'd have to order some. His conversation completed, he turned and hurled toward me on his wheeled chair, stopping just inches before careening into me.

"Sorry. Now where were we? Oh, yes, you're here to apply for an internship. Tell me, why do you think our association would be a symbiotic one?"

As professionally as I could, I explained my love of writing, my desire to enter the communications field and the hope that such a position at CHOC would be a learning experience for me as well as a chance to relieve him from some of the responsibility for the hospital's publications.

"I've brought along some of the articles I've written for the college paper," I said, handing him my stringbook and adding that I'd been editing such publications since my junior high school days.

Vick, as he insisted I call him, quickly flipped through the pages of my scrapbook, offering praise for a story's lead here, commenting on an activity I'd covered there—then abruptly slammed the book shut.

"Well, unless someone shows up later today with the writing skills of Mark Twain, the speaking ability of Charles Darrow and the looks of Raquel Welch, you've got the job. Can you start Monday?"

Vick and I had established a wonderful rapport from the beginning. I considered him my mentor—and my friend—and through the next few years, I called him often for professional advice and met him for lunch whenever either of us was in the other's corporate neighborhoods.

Now that I was single, Vick had begun showing interest in seeing me during times other than business hours.

I snapped myself out of my reverie. "Girls, Vick's going to be here any minute. Here's the phone number of the people having the party. Now, you call if there's any problem, okay?"

Kathy smiled and hugged me. "Don't worry, we'll be fine. And Mom? You look really cute in my new blue dress."

We laughed. Nothing in my closet had been quite right. My wardrobe reflected my business image. I didn't even have a social image and couldn't remember the last time I'd been to a party. What luck to have a daughter who was not only the same size but generous enough to share.

Suddenly I realized that Meri was not in the room. I walked into her bedroom and found her sitting on her bed, sniffling to hold back the tears. I knelt down and took her solemn little face in my hands.

"Momma, you're not going to get married are you?"

"Oh, Meri. Is that what's bothering you? Believe me, marriage is the farthest thing from my mind right now. Vick is just a very dear friend, honey."

I stood and pulled my younger daughter up with me. "Meri, this is the first date I've had in more than 16 years—and you've already got me married."

I smiled. "You just wait until you have a date. I'm going to cry and ask you if you're eloping."

We both fell onto the bed and began to giggle at that. The doorbell rang, interrupting our laughter, and my eyes sobered and met Meri's.

"Hurry, Momma. There he is. You don't want to be late for your first date, do you?"

I kissed my 12 year old and held her tight for a minute more. I loved her so much.

I walked to the front door and looked through the peep hole. There he was. Regardless of my words to the contrary, and despite my resolve not to become emotionally involved, I felt my heart begin to pound.

Vick Knight was one special man.

11

I lay on the sweet-smelling carpet of new grass and slowly opened my eyes. Above me the sprouting branches of a sycamore waved in the breeze, as if conducting a silent symphony to springtime. How I loved this time of the year. Everywhere I looked there were signs of new life. Tiny shoots pushing up through the sun-warmed soil. Chartreuse leaves dotting the city's trees. Sparrows and blackbirds swooping everywhere to pick up a tiny twig here, a piece of string there.

I smiled. I was beginning to feel the nesting instinct myself. Granted, single life did have its advantages. But I missed the sense of family. You know. Papa bear, mommy bear, baby bears. I missed belonging, not *to* someone, but *with* someone. I missed . . .

"Ouch." My meditation was brought abruptly to a halt by the sting of a Frisbee skidding to a halt alongside my ear.

"Get up, lazy. If I can cook dinner, the least you can do is stay awake long enough to eat it."

Vick offered me his hand and helped me to my feet. With the warmer weather and the longer daylight hours, we often met at the park near my condo for a picnic in the evening. Kathy and Meri loved these outings, too, and always brought along their shoe skates to take advantage of the smooth sloping sidewalks meandering through the area.

Tonight Vick had brought along ballpark franks to sizzle on one of the barbecue pits and, from the looks of them, they were going to turn into charcoal themselves if we didn't quickly get them off the grill and into the buns I'd brought.

"See if you can find the kids. I'll take over here," I said.

I didn't want to tell Vick that I probably couldn't walk to the crest of the hill and back without struggling for breath. I had been experiencing some difficulty breathing today for some reason. I hadn't kept my asthma a secret from him, but I didn't make a big issue of it either. He knew, of course, that I avoided restaurants, and why, but picnic suppers like the one we were having tonight more than made up for not dining out—and I certainly didn't want to scare him off by going to a restaurant with him and ending up in the emergency room.

I watched Vick fondly as he hurried to the top of the hill and began to wave his arms frantically to get the girls' attention. To friend and mentor, I now added the words lover and confidante. What more could I want in a man?

I turned to the little picnic table under the tree and quickly prepared it for the hungry trio now running toward me. Chips, pickles, fresh fruit, soft drinks—and hot dogs. A meal fit for a king—or at the very least a Knight.

Later that evening we snuggled on the couch content in each other's company. After our return from the park, we'd helped the girls with their homework, and they'd talked Vick into a trip to 31 Flavors for triple-decker rocky road ice cream cones. Now that they were finally tucked away for the night, we could enjoy some quiet time to hug and cuddle and share with each other the happenings of our days.

"What about Easter?" I asked. "Will you be able to join us at my parents for dinner?"

"I'd like to sweetie. Let me see what I can work out."

I sighed. If there's anything I'd learned in the past year, it was that divorce could certainly make holidays chaotic. Jerry wanted Kathy and Meri to spend the day with him and his new girlfriend, his family wanted the girls to attend services with them, and my mom and dad had asked us to have dinner at their house. Vick's life was equally as complicated, with parents and sisters and married children all wanting him to drop by also. It was impossible to please everyone.

I hugged my teddy-bear of a man. "I know. If we get up early enough Easter Sunday, we can make the rounds and see everyone."

I began counting on my fingers and then took off my shoes and began tabulating on my toes as well. "Let's see. Fourteen stops between the hours of 10 a.m. and 6 p.m. Allowing for travel time, we could spend 10 or 15 minutes with everyone on the list."

Vick grinned at me. "You're weird, you know that? But you're lovable."

He kissed me and held me gently in his arms. "Tell your mom and dad we'll have dinner with them—then maybe we can drive into Hollywood for dessert with my folks."

Easter Sunday dawned bright and clear and I hurried around the house opening all the drapes to welcome in the beautiful sunny day. On the dining room table sat two floppy straw hats, turned upside down with the crowns filled with bright green plastic grass. I had put them there the night before and now I rushed to place chocolate rabbits, marshmallow chicks and colorful hard-boiled eggs atop the grass before the girls awakened. I knew they felt they were too old for visits from the Easter Bunny, but I also knew they'd be pleased with all the goodies—and the new spring hats.

They were.

"Yum. I love these things," Kathy said, stuffing her mouth with chocolate eggs and jelly beans.

Meri dumped the contents of her makeshift basket on the table so that she could try on her new "Easter bonnet."

"Oh, Momma. This is the cutest straw hat I ever saw." She ran to the mirror to admire herself, oblivious to the strands of plastic grass clinging to her hair.

"Okay, you two. Let's get breakfast and our showers over with pronto. Vick will be here to pick us up in an hour. We're due at Grandmother's and Granddaddy's at one."

Our 45-minute drive into Lakewood turned into a time for fun and games. Even the most mundane activities could prove entertaining when Vick was around. We played word games as we zoomed over the Orange County freeways and were just finishing up a lively version of "Gossip" when we pulled up in front of the house where I'd grown up so many years before.

Mother was in the kitchen putting final touches on the ham and mixing up Meri's favorite fruit salad—"Purple Passion," a combination of whipped cream, Bing cherries, almonds and miniature marshmallows. Daddy had set up two long tables on the screened-in back porch. It was such a pleasant day that we were going to eat our meal there.

"I've brought along some of my homemade wine," said Vick, holding out the bottle of Johannisberg Riesling. "I'll just store it in the refrigerator for now."

Mother caught my eye and wrinkled her nose. She and Daddy didn't drink wine and neither did my sister, Jan, nor her husband. We might have talked Aunt Helen into sipping some, but she'd just found out she was diabetic. And Uncle Rod thought wine was a sissy drink.

Poor Vick. He'd wanted so much to provide something special for our meal. And he was so proud of that wine. He and his father, Vick Sr., had enjoyed their roles as home vintners for some time, turning out 500 bottles a year in "Big Dad's" converted garage in West Hollywood. They even had special labels printed and affixed to their bottles and friends were always pleased to receive gifts from "The Westside Grapist."

Well, most friends, anyway. My family certainly didn't consist of wine connoisseurs. And, to tell the truth, I'd always avoided this particular variety of grape juice myself.

I'd often told my doctors I seemed to wheeze more after a glass of wine, and they had said it was because of the histamine in this alcoholic beverage.

"Vicko, I'll join you in a glass of that wine right now."

It was against my better judgment, but if I could help my friend polish off the bottle before dinner, he wouldn't have to put up with the rest of my family turning up their noses when he offered them some.

We sat out on the glider on the back porch, rocking gently and sipping the vino. Actually it was the best wine I'd ever tasted, and I told Vick so. I had to admit I'd never had white wine before. I'd always chosen red, assuming from its color that it would be sweet. In the past, I'd filled my glass with part wine and part 7-Up just to avoid making a face when I swallowed. This stuff was really good, though.

"I know your dad doesn't have a vineyard in Hollywood," I said. "Where do you get the supplies you need to make all this wine?"

"We have various wineries that are willing to sell us the grapes we need," began Vick, warming to one of his favorite subjects.

I felt my lungs tighten. Oh, no. This wine was going to make me wheeze, too. Vick's voice rambled on, regaling me with stories on wine-making as I reached into my purse and felt for the inhaler I used to relax my constricted airways. I smiled at Vick and pretended to listen intently as I squirted the inhaler's contents into my lungs and held my breath as the directions instructed.

Oh, Jesus. My hands were beginning to itch. I grabbed my purse, made some excuse and, walking as calmly as possible, entered my parents' bedroom and shut the door. I pulled down my slacks and sat on the edge of the bed, reaching into my handbag for my adrenalin kit.

The attack seemed worse than any I could remember. My ears began to ring and my whole body felt as if it were on fire. I wasn't breathing in enough air to even wheeze. Not caring if I bruised myself or not, I jammed the needle into my leg and lay back on the bed.

It wasn't helping. Oh, God. It wasn't helping.

I again drew up some of the serum into the small needle and gave myself a second injection, trying to fight off the feeling of faintness that was coming over me.

I needed help. Now.

Standing up, I began to walk toward the door while pulling up my pants. I caught sight of myself in the bedroom mirror and hardly recognized the face I saw. It was gray and the eyes were huge and staring. I looked like a corpse.

I moaned. This is it. This time I'm not going to make it. I reached the back porch and everything seemed to be happening in slow motion.

My mother was the first to notice me. "Oh, my Lord." She jumped up out of her chair and put her hands to her cheeks. Kathy and Meri began to whimper. Vick was at my side in an instant.

"Russ, is there a hospital close by?" he asked my dad.

Following Vick's quick commands, my dad rushed to get my purse since it contained all my emergency medical information and then helped drag me out the front door. I was still able to put one foot in front of the other, but it was the strength of the men on either side of me holding my arms that propelled me to the car.

Once inside and on our way, Daddy gave directions to Vick and kept patting my shoulder. "Hang on, kid. Hang on."

Daddy's voice sounded far away.

I'm dying. I know I'm dying. I need another shot. My hand reached ever so slowly for the glove compartment and the adrenalin kit I kept there. Still trying to control my panic, I pulled up the leg of my black pants as far as I could to prepare my thigh for a third needle. But this time I couldn't make my hands obey. I felt the syringe drop from my fingers and slumped unconscious against the car door.

12

An eerie calm engulfed me, and I suddenly was unaware of any physical distress. I knew I was dying, but the thought was not an anguished one any longer. I felt myself float above my oxygen-deprived body and almost casually observed the scene around me.

Vick was leaning forward, the knuckles of his hands white from his fierce grip on the steering wheel. His foot pushed the accelerator to the floor as we sped over the residential streets toward the small neighborhood hospital.

"How much farther?"

Daddy's voice shook in reply. "It's the first right after the intersection."

The light turned red as our car approached, but we propelled through it anyway, our horn blaring and Vick swearing under his breath.

Poor Vick. He's so upset that I'm dying. He'll miss me.

The brakes squealed as Vick applied them sharply to make the right turn. We pulled up in front of the emergency ward, the little station wagon careening over the curb before being brought abruptly to a halt. Leaving the motor running, Vick jumped out and ran around to open the passenger door. Daddy reached forward from the back seat to keep me from falling onto the pavement.

Still hovering above, I watched my loved ones struggle with my rag-doll body as they pulled it from the car.

Dear Daddy. Sweet Vick. Don't worry. I'm in no pain.

With their hands under my armpits, they balanced me between them and dragged me through the swinging doors.

"She's in shock. Get adrenalin. STAT." Vick's experience as a hospital administrator gave him an advantage, and he was able to speak authoritatively in a language the emergency staff understood.

A doctor, his white coat flapping behind him as he ran, hurried toward us and helped Vick lift my unconscious body onto the examination table. My complexion was chalky, and my lips were blue.

Continuing to observe the flurry of activity, I saw the doctor and two nurses quickly ready a syringe with epinephrine and apply an oxygen mask to my nose and mouth. Daddy, who couldn't stand it when my sisters or I skinned our knees when we were little, left the room, saying he'd take care of the car.

Vick stood at the head of the narrow, metal table. His face was a study in agony, his normally animated expression now drawn and pinched in grief. His tortured eyes never left my face, and his strong hand squeezed my limp one as if, by sheer will, he could help me hang on to my waning life.

I felt myself float even higher and the tranquility surrounding me was such a contrast to the frenzied scene below, a scene I viewed with detachment.

Suddenly I heard Vick sob. "Sweet Caroline. Sweet Caroline."

I can't leave him. I just can't. Our time together is just beginning. And the girls. My Kathy. Little Meri. They need me . . . .

I opened my eyes and tried to focus but the bright ceiling lights faded in and out, and Vick's face swam above me. My nose hurt, and I reached up with my free hand and felt tubes running into my nostrils. Oxygen. An IV drip, drip, dripped into a vein in my extended right arm, and Vick still clung to my hand.

"I love you," he said, his voice trembling.

I nodded, too exhausted to make any other reply.

The effects of so much adrenalin and the knowledge that I had once again almost died overwhelmed me, and I began to cry.

Vick gently wiped the tears from my cheeks and bent to kiss my forehead.

"Don't cry. You're going to be okay now. I wasn't about to let you get away from me."

My body involuntarily took a long, deep breath, and I felt my strength returning. The corners of my mouth turned up, and I looked at my cherished friend and lover.

"You're in trouble now," I whispered.

"What do you mean by that?" He turned his head and leaned his ear closer to my lips.

"There's a Chinese proverb that says if you save someone from death, you're responsible for that person for the rest of your life."

Vick stood up and smiled down at me, his blue eyes twinkling. "Well," he said softly, "I guess I'm stuck with you then."

Within an hour I was breathing easily and the nurse began disconnecting me from the wires, tubes and needles invading my body. Vick, who had never left my side, took my arm and led me from the room.

Daddy stood up as we entered the small lobby. His face was ashen, and he hugged me tight. Holding out my handbag toward me, he began to apologize.

"I couldn't find your medical cards, so I dumped everything in your purse onto the table. I'm afraid it's a mess now."

I took my dad's hand. It was still shaking.

"Come on, Daddy. Let's go home. I'm hungry."

And, I was. Mother's ham was delicious and the rest of the meal equally as good. My family couldn't believe I felt like staying, let alone eating. The dinner time conversation was punctuated with laughter as everyone attempted to alleviate the tension of the previous hours. Throughout the afternoon, each person there felt compelled to touch me, to stroke my arm or to give me a quick hug. It was as if they needed to make certain that I was really there and really all right. I found myself in the position of comforter—an ironic twist since I was the one who had almost died.

It wasn't until that evening, after the girls had gone to bed that I finally let my emotions flow. Vick listened as I relived the terrifying events, tightening his embrace as I recounted my out-of-body experience and my decision to return to my torpid form rather than accept the floating peacefulness and the promise it held.

I sighed and finally fell silent.

Though I had told Vick of my occurrences of anaphylaxis, this was the first one he had experienced and I knew he was still shaken.

"What can we do to keep this from ever happening again?"

"I wish I knew. This is the ninth time it's happened in seven years."

Releasing myself from his arms, I sat upright on the couch. "You know, this is the first time I wasn't in a restaurant . . . ."

I bolted to my feet. "The wine. It's got to be something in the wine."

I turned to Vick. "Whatever I'm allergic to has got to be in the wine you and your dad made."

"But there's nothing but grapes in wine."

"That's what I've always thought, too, but check anyway, would you? Maybe he sneaks something in while you're not looking."

The following day, Vick called me at the office with the information I'd been waiting for since my speculation the night before.

"You're right," he said. "There was something in the wine. Dad uses some stuff called potassium metabisulfite to wash his bottles and to help control fermentation."

"Meta what?"

He spelled the long chemical name for me. "Dad was really mortified about what happened to you yesterday. He was on the verge of tears when I told him there was a possibility our wine sent you to the emergency ward."

"Listen," I said. "You call him back and tell him I love him. This is the first really substantial clue I've ever had. I've got to go. I'm going to call Scripps."

As usual, Dr. Stevens' secretary took my name and number and said she'd have him call me back. I was so excited I couldn't concentrate on the magazine article I was supposed to be writing, so I grabbed a phone book, called a local wine supply store and was told that potassium metabisulfite could be purchased there.

It was almost 4 p.m. when Dr. Stevens returned my call. I excitedly told him of the events of the previous day and asked if I could make an appointment for a "challenge test."

"We'll need more than just an hour or two appointment to do this right," my doctor said. "You'd better plan on coming down and admitting yourself as an in-patient for two or three days."

I told him I'd let him know when I could do so, then hung up and spun around and around in my chair. It was wonderful to have a doctor who really listened. A doctor who believed that, as a patient, I should be as educated as possible about my disease. A doctor who welcomed my input and my theories.

From now on I would never retain the services of a doctor who was not willing to treat me as more than a lung—or a leg—or an eye—that needed his ministrations. After all, patients actually hire their physicians. Most people wouldn't think of engaging the services of a babysitter, a real estate agent or even a plumber without some kind of a contract or understanding. Yet these same people so often put their most precious possession—their health—into the hands of a doctor and assume that as long as he has that medical degree hanging on the wall, he is competent to give them the care they need. I learned the hard way that this is certainly the wrong way to approach the issue of finding a doctor.

I now knew that it is vitally important to know a physician's philosophy before committing to his care—especially an allergist. Is the doctor open to patient input? Is he willing to discuss new theories and treatments? How does he feel about the somewhat controversial but upcoming field of clinical ecology that recognizes that a broad array of environmental chemicals can cause allergy and disease? The doctor-patient relationship, I'd decided, should definitely be a working partnership. I was glad I'd established such a partnership with Dr. Stevens.

I made arrangements for Kathy and Meri to stay with their dad, told my department head I'd need three days off and left for La Jolla the following Wednesday, stopping by the wine supply store on my way to purchase a small packet of the chemical in question. It certainly looked innocuous enough. It could have been sugar or salt judging from its looks. Could it really be deadly, I wondered as I drove the scenic coastal route toward the south.

Scripps Clinic had grown tremendously since my first visit there, and it was now housed in a beautiful new building high on a cliff. Despite the expansion, members of the staff maintained a personal touch with their patients, and I was greeted with exuberant hellos from my friends in the division of allergy.

"This is it. I'm sure of it!" I waved the little plastic package of potassium metabisulfite in the air, then tossed it to Dr. Stevens.

"Well, we'll soon find out, won't we?" The doctor smiled and told me to go ahead and check into my room. "I'll be up shortly to discuss the study with you."

I entered my private room and unpacked the couple of nightgowns and the toiletries I'd brought along, then opened my briefcase and set it on the desk in the corner. I'd brought along some work I had to finish.

Deadlines on corporate publications don't wait just because the editor takes a few days off.

Minutes later, Dr. Stevens dropped in and explained the next day's activities.

"We'll be conducting this challenge in a strictly scientific manner," he said. "If your hunch is right, we want your reaction documented so the medical community will accept it."

He explained that, in a double-blind study, neither the patient nor the staff knew the contents of the pill being given. None of us would know tomorrow if I were receiving placebos or capsules filled with the chemical I'd brought.

"I guess I can see why you wouldn't want me to know what I'm ingesting, but why shouldn't you and the nurses know?"

Dr. Stevens smiled and sat down. He knew I'd become the kind of patient who could ask questions for hours. "I can see I might as well get comfortable," he said. He crossed his long legs and leaned back in the chair.

"There are those who believe that the nurse giving you the pill might convey by a look or through body language that she's offering you the suspected allergen. And that might trigger a psychological response," he explained. "The pills you'll receive are all numbered, and only the pharmacist who prepared them knows the code."

I didn't think I was the type to react emotionally, but I'd cooperate and do it any way they wanted. If I were allergic to potassium metabisulfite, I didn't want my discovery discounted by a doubting medical profession.

The next morning I arrived in the allergy department's testing lab at nine o'clock. I'd brought along a novel I'd been wanting to read to help pass the time. I knew from other challenges I'd had at the Clinic that a long day stretched ahead.

Before the testing began, Pat, the technician, recorded my lung function score to tabulate how much air I could expend in one breath. Similar tests would be conducted a half hour after each pill I was given to gauge my reaction, if any, to whatever that capsule contained.

The day passed slowly. Take a pill. Wait 30 minutes. Blow in the machine. Gulp, wait, blow. Gulp, wait, blow.

Nothing happened.

I sat on the uncomfortable little cot in the bare little testing room all day, waiting for a response. None came. At 5 p.m. I returned to my room, discouraged because, once again, it appeared I had collided with a brick wall.

That evening after dinner and the six o'clock news, I changed into my bed clothes and slipped between the covers of the hospital bed. There was no reason I should be so tired—I'd done nothing but sit and read all day. Nonetheless, a weariness—more mental than physical—enveloped me and I soon fell into a restless sleep.

My tossing and turning was interrupted by the loud buzzing of the telephone next to my bed, and I picked up the receiver to hear Vick's concerned voice.

"Hi, Sweet Caroline. You've been on my mind every minute today. What's happening down there?"

"Nothing. Absolutely nothing." I had been so upbeat and hopeful when I'd left him the day before, but now I was unable to mask the frustration I felt about the day's testing.

"Oh, Vick. I guess I shouldn't let myself get so excited every time I hear about a new medicine or every time I manufacture a new theory about controlling this damn problem of mine.

"But this time I really thought I'd found the answer . . . ."

My voice trailed off, and I sat there holding the phone to my ear and fighting back the tears. When was I ever going to stop looking for a miracle?

Vick tried to be reassuring. "Hey, don't give up yet. Maybe you'll get the answer you're looking for tomorrow."

"Sure, Vick, maybe tomorrow . . . ."

The next day I rose early and was back in the four-foot by eight-foot testing room at nine o'clock, ready for an instant replay of the day before. I had given myself a pep talk in the shower that morning and had philosophically told myself that, as long as there were new drugs and new theories to try, there was still hope.

At least I've had a chance to catch up on my reading, I thought, settling down once again in the cramped little room and turning the pages of Herman Wouk's *War and Remembrance.*

I had been through the gulp, wait, blow routine twice when I noticed I was absent-mindedly balancing the cumbersome book in my right hand so that I could rub the palm of my left hand on the edge of the table in front of me.

My hands were itching!

I shouted to the technician. "Pat, I'm having a reaction."

"It's about time something happened around here," she said, teasing me. "Come on out and blow for me."

By the time I had walked around the corner my chest had tightened so much that it felt as if it were being constricted by an iron band. A puff of air was all I was able to expend into the machine, and I was so short of breath I couldn't speak.

Pat was immediately aware of the dangers and called for Dr. Stevens as she helped me to a large examination chair and released the back to place me in a prone position. A generous dose of adrenalin and immediate relief from a respirator kept me from reaching the coma-stage that so often accompanied my anaphylactic reactions. Within ten minutes my plunging blood pressure was stabilized and I was breathing normally—and on my own.

Dr. Stevens and the other members of the staff began to gather around me. Everyone was beaming and patting each other on the back. Dr. Stevens sat on a stool next to me and smiled his boyish grin.

"Well, Sherlock, we've checked with the pharmacist. You were right."

I was still unnerved by the experience, which had been equally as frightening as the others I'd had despite the controlled environment.

That didn't stop me, though, from faking a British accent and returning my doctor's quip.

"Potassium metabisulfite, I presume."

13

I was Madame Curie, Philip Marlowe and Sam Spade all rolled into one. I'd made an important discovery—solved a mystery that even the best doctors at one of the most prestigious medical institutions in the world could not.

Fluffing up the pillow on the hospital bed, I fell back into its comfortable softness and waited for Dr. Stevens to arrive with my release form. I smiled and continued my daydreaming. Maybe I'd end up in the encyclopedia someday. Best of all, I finally had an answer—finally knew what was causing my life-threatening episodes. And just in time. I'd experienced anaphylaxis nine times. Even a cat had only nine lives. How could I expect to be any luckier?

Dr. Stevens walked into my room and squeezed my shoulder. "How are you feeling?"

"Fantastic. I can't believe we've finally found the culprit."

Dr. Stevens' smile faded and, removing his glasses, he massaged the bridge of his nose. "I just wish I knew more about this substance. Potassium metabisulfite is a form of sulfur dioxide, but I'm not sure of its uses."

Swinging my legs off the bed and sitting on the edge of the mattress, I looked at Dr. Stevens. "Don't be so glum. We know what to fight now. We'll just find out how the stuff is used. I'm getting pretty good at this detective work," I said none too modestly.

After all, wasn't I Madame Curie, Philip Marlowe and Sam Spade all rolled into one?

My first item of business when I returned to work the following Monday was to place a call to my company's quality control manager. The firm I worked for owned a large chain of restaurants, and the commissary that supplied the 300 outlets was located adjacent to the corporate headquarters where I had my office.

Don McNally called me back within minutes. "Hey, Carolyn, how are you? I've been meaning to call you and thank you for the nice article you wrote about the meat processing department in the last company magazine."

"You're welcome, Don. It was a fun story to write. Everyone's interested in reading about a machine that can produce 18,000 hamburger patties an hour."

We exchanged pleasantries for a few more minutes before I took a deep breath and plunged into my topic of concern.

"Listen, Don, have you ever heard of a chemical called potassium metabisulfite?"

"Sure. Everyone in the food industry knows about sulfites—are you planning to do an article on anti-oxidants?"

I grabbed a pencil and some paper out of my drawer and quickly scrawled the word "anti-oxidant" across the yellow pad. "No, I'm not writing an article, just doing some personal research. What can you tell me about sulfites?"

"Well, in general, sulfiting agents are used to keep foods from turning color. You know how fruits and vegetables, like apples and potatoes, turn brown when they're cut? Sulfiting agents keep that from happening."

My pen flew over the paper as I attempted to take down the manager's every word.

"Don, is it ever used on salads?"

"Oh, sure. Restaurants use it on almost all salad vegetables. I've been told it can keep a head of lettuce fresh and crisp for as long as a year."

I gasped, but Don was so intent on his subject that he seemed not to notice. "Sulfites are the major ingredient in products like 'Sta-Fresh,' 'White All' and 'Potato White.' The stuff's amazing. The restaurant industry relies on it to keep lots of its menu items looking appetizing. Oh, no. Hey, Carolyn, can I get back to you? One of the machines just stopped."

I thanked him, replaced the receiver and stared at the telephone. I couldn't believe what I'd heard. The answer had been right under my nose the whole time, but I hadn't known where to look.

I immediately picked up the phone once again and dialed Dr. Stevens, who for a change was able to take my call right away. I told him what I'd learned that morning.

He sounded impressed that I'd already discovered so much. "Good work, Carolyn. I'll get off a letter to the FDA today and find out just how extensively this stuff is used. And, listen friend, stay out of restaurants, okay?"

We both laughed. That's one directive I didn't need. I couldn't remember the last time I'd eaten a meal out anyway.

The following week, I received a copy of the letter Dr. Stevens had sent to the Food and Drug Administration, addressed to the Division of Drug Experience, Office of Biometrics and Epidemiology.

Dear Sirs:

We have recently documented an anaphylactic reaction in one of our patients after ingestion of potassium metabisulfite. I'm aware that this drug is used in a compound called "White All" for the preparation of lettuce in certain restaurants and that it is also used in the wine industry, presumably as a preservative. I would be interested in finding out whether this compound has generalized approval for use in human beings or whether it is restricted to certain food stuffs. It would be very helpful in the management of this patient's anaphylaxis to have that information.

Within a month, we had the following reply:

Dear Dr. Stevens:

This is in reply to your letter of April 30, 1979, inquiring about potassium metabisulfite. I contacted the Bureau of Foods who informed me that potassium metabisulfite is considered a safe anti-oxidant and my be used in foods that do not contain vitamin B_1, as it deactivates that vitamin. It also cannot be used in meats. The person I spoke with felt information may be available about food stuffs containing this chemical. I have referred your letter to the Bureau of Foods so that they may send this information to you.

The information from the Bureau of Foods arrived shortly thereafter. Titled an "Evaluation of the Health Aspects of Sulfiting Agents as Food Ingredients," the fifteen-page report concluded that there was no evidence that sulfiting agents were a hazard to the public. The chemicals were considered "GRAS," generally recognized as safe, and as such were exempt from the premarketing clearances required for food additives.

Safe? How could sulfites be considered safe when they had almost killed me nine times? Cyclamates had been taken off the market. Saccharin had been proclaimed hazardous. How many times had I read about foods being banned merely because it was *suspected* that they caused health problems. I was angry and frustrated. Did a rat have to die before the government would reconsider the safety of a product?

The paper from the FDA was very vague about the use of sulfites but mentioned wines and light-colored fruits, such as apples, pears, peaches and apricots, as the types of foods in which the chemical could be found. Yet a trip to the grocery store revealed no mention of the food additive in these fruits except when dried.

"Evidently the FDA considers sulfiting agents so safe that it doesn't even require labeling," said Dr. Stevens as he and I discussed the issue in his office the next month.

"Well I'm not going to eat any more processed foods unless they state that they're preserved with ascorbic or citric acid," I said. "My theory is that I'm ingesting enough sulfites in the foods I eat to keep me chronically asthmatic. Then when I'm exposed to a large amount of it, as I am in restaurants, I go into anaphylactic shock."

"I think you're absolutely right, Carolyn. And I'm concerned about the fact that you're living in such a smoggy area. Sulfur dioxide is a major component of air pollution, you know."

Yes, I knew. I was being inundated with SO_2. The condominium I had so proudly bought a year and a half before was bounded on three sides by freeways and was on the corridor to the Santa Ana Canyon. The car exhaust I was exposed to daily was suffocating, and all the smog from Los Angeles and Orange Counties swept right past my nose as it funneled through the pass to end up trapped by the mountains in San Bernardino. To make matters worse, I worked in one of the smoggiest cities in the area.

More and more frequently I found myself waking at 5 a.m. and stumbling to the bathroom for a shot of adrenalin to start my day. By the time the unsuspecting girls awakened at six, I was breathing easily. And by the time I arrived at the office at eight, no one would ever have guessed that I had been on the verge of hospitalization just three hours before. Once the adrenalin had worn off, high doses of cortisone had taken over and helped my lungs function well all day long.

I was also relying more and more on my portable breathing machine. I had bought the little table-model Intermittent Positive Pressure Breathing Machine (IPPB) when my asthma had first begun in the early 1970s, but had kept it hidden away most of the time. Seeing it sitting on a counter or desk was a constant reminder of my illness—and something I didn't want to advertise. However, I now began to drag it out of the closet more and more often, using it before I went to work, as added insurance for a wheeze-free day, as well as when I got home from the office so that I could enjoy my evenings and any activities they might bring.

One morning I opened the refrigerator to get the inhalant medication and saline that I used and set up my machine to take the normal 15-minute treatment. I usually read the morning paper during this time, but it had not yet arrived so, for lack of anything better to do, I began reading the cereal boxes I had set out for the girls' breakfast and then glanced at the label on the Bronkosol that had been prescribed for my IPPB.

My eyes widened at what I saw, and I spit the long rubber tube out of my mouth.

Sodium bisulfite.

The drug was preserved with sodium bisulfite!

Oh, my God.

I ran to my medicine cabinet and grabbed the literature from the boxes of medications I always kept in ready supply. Three others were also preserved with my allergen.

I couldn't believe it. The drugs that were supposed to control my asthma were adding to my problem. The implications of the discovery overpowered me and I walked into my bedroom and lay on the bed. I felt like a female Job from the Bible story I'd read as a child. One more tribulation had been added for me to suffer. As if I didn't have enough already. The frequent doses of adrenalin were adversely affecting my heart, I knew. And a trip to the ophthalmologist had recently confirmed my fears that my eyesight was failing because of cortisone-induced cataracts. The extremely potent drug was also causing my joints to deteriorate, making it very painful for me to continue my daily walking exercises. If I continued to rely on this powerful medication, I knew I'd end up with additional health problems. That's just what I needed—to be a blind, crippled asthmatic!

I got up and began dressing for work. Once I got to the office, I'd make a call to the Clinic and tell Dr. Stevens of my most recent finding.

My doctor was as astounded as I, but was able to prescribe substitute drugs for those I could no longer take.

"Never take a drug from any doctor without having him check that medication in his Physician's Desk Reference," he cautioned me, referring to a large text filled with information about every prescription drug on the market. He also encouraged me to make an appointment to see him the following week then said goodbye, urging me to keep my chin up.

"Carolyn, you've got to consider leaving the area," Dr. Stevens advised me when I saw him the next Monday.

"Oh, Dr. Stevens, if you had your way, I'd move to a log cabin in Wyoming or Montana and grow my own food," I said, trying to be flip but sounding defensive instead. "I have two daughters to support, and college is just a year away for the older one. I can't just quit my job and move away. I wish it were that simple."

As I drove home from La Jolla after my appointment that afternoon, I barely noticed the beautiful ocean view that usually captivated me. I'd been naive to assume that discovering my asthma's cause would give me a new lease on life. I laughed bitterly. I'd actually thought that all I'd have to do to be cured was to avoid the chemical that caused my problem. Oh, I was glad to know what to fight, but the chemical was so widely used in foods and so prevalent in the air I breathed that it was impossible to escape. In fact, my problems had begun in Huntington Beach—just a mile upwind from the largest emitter of SO_2 in the county. Foggy conditions kept the sulfur pollution from escaping, and the ocean breezes brought the contaminated air right through my neighborhood.

I felt defeated and afraid. Then in a mood swing that surprised even me, I was filled with rage.

How dare the FDA authorize the almost indiscriminate use of such a dangerous substance?

How dare food processors use chemicals in their products and not inform consumers?

How dare restaurants saturate their menu items with this additive just to make their food appear more appetizing?

Angry tears blinded my eyes and I brushed them away as I traveled the road through San Clemente. I pounded the steering wheel. When people ordered salads or vegetables and fruit platters in restaurants, they thought they were doing something good for their bodies. They had no idea they were eating a potentially dangerous chemical.

I continued to fume as I drove up the coast toward my home. I had always assumed that restaurant food was even more fresh than that I served at home. After all, I shopped just once a week, so food often sat in my refrigerator for several days before being eaten. But restaurants received their produce every day—there was no need to preserve it. The restaurant industry must use sulfiting agents for cosmetic purposes only—and that shouldn't be allowed. That was deceiving the public. There ought to be a law.

14

Still livid, I pulled my silver sports car into the parking lot of the condominium complex and into the space reserved for me. I slammed the car door shut, stomped up the walk and burst into the house. The girls were setting the table and giggling. One look into the kitchen told me why.

Vick was standing at the stove wearing an apron and a chef's hat that made him at least two feet taller. He was stirring a huge pot, and a delicious smell was permeating the room.

"Hi, sweetie. I knew you'd probably be tired after your long drive home from the Clinic, so I decided to come over and cook my specialty for you."

"He's making fettuccine, Mom," Kathy informed me.

"And Italian sausage and peppers, too," Meri added.

Now here was a man who knew how to dissipate my anger in a hurry. I loved Italian food—and knowing I wouldn't have to cook dinner made me feel better immediately.

"Who ever told you the way to a woman's heart was through her stomach?" I teased, accepting his kiss.

Later that evening when the girls were upstairs doing their homework, I shared my earlier anger with Vick, telling him how discouraged I felt about my inability to do anything about the problem.

"How many people have died because they aren't as lucky as I?" My voice raised. "How many people are in the emergency room right now being told they've choked on a piece of lettuce? I've got to find a way to do something about this. I've just got to."

Vick smiled at me and touched my cheek. "If anyone can find a way to make them ban this stuff, it's you," he said. "And all I can say is I'd hate to be the director of the FDA when you come storming through the door."

We laughed together and then both became quiet as we hugged, watching the flames leaping in the tiny, free-standing fireplace. I felt the tension leave my body and, pushing away the exasperation of the day, I was aware only of the strong, loving arms embracing me.

We were jolted out of our peaceful mood by Kathy and Meri who, having finished their studies, decided to join us on the hearth. Both girls were taller than I now, and they had grown in beauty as well as height. They jockeyed for position, trying to get as close to us and the warmth of the fire as possible.

"We need a bigger fireplace," Kathy said.

Vick stood up and stretched. "Here, take my place. It's time for me to get on home, anyway. But, I've got a deal for all of you. I've got a big mailing I've got to get out for the hospital and I need some help."

"We'll help you, Vicko," Meri said.

"Good. I'll bring it over tomorrow night, then—and we'll have a contest to see who can stuff and lick the most envelopes, okay?"

The girls loved the idea. I sat there smiling and watched Meri's eyes light up. "What's the prize, Vicko?"

"A giant pizza—and the winner can choose what goes on top."

The girls jumped up and hugged Vick. I wasn't the only one who loved Italian food.

The next evening, the four of us sat around the dining room table surrounded by boxes of stationery and envelopes.

"Now here's what we've got to do," Vick said. "Each of these letters has to be folded into thirds and stuffed into an envelope, then licked shut."

"How many are there?" asked Kathy.

"Only 1500."

Both girls groaned. "Let's work in teams," Meri suggested. "I'll be your partner, Momma."

"On your marks, get set, go." Kathy and Vick were on one side of the table and Meri and I on the other as we began folding, stuffing and licking. We laughed and joked as we worked and tried different methods to see which would get the job done fastest.

Vick stuck his tongue out. "Here, Kathy, I'll be a licking machine." Kathy stuffed an envelope then ran it along Vick's tongue to seal it. We all laughed. Leave it to Vick to make even the most ordinary task into a game.

About 15 minutes into the job, I began coughing and wheezing. Damn it. I'd taken my pills. Why was I having an asthma attack? Stupid lungs, not now. Not when we're having such a good time.

I decided to practice some "pursed lip" breathing, exercises I'd learned that not only helped build an asthmatic's lung function and stamina, but which I'd also found a helpful technique to use during an attack, because it kept up the air pressure in the bronchial tubes and helped move stale, trapped air out.

Continuing to keep my hands busy at the task, I tried to nonchalantly inhale as much air as I could through my nose and exhale it slowly through my puckered lips.

This time it didn't seem to be working for me, however. I tried to ignore the tightness in my chest and continued the routine Meri and I had established, with her folding letters and me stuffing them into envelopes and licking them shut.

Finally the rattling sound I was making became so loud that Vick and the girls looked at me with concern.

"Do you want me to get your inhaler, Mom?" I nodded and Kathy dashed up the stairs and found it. Vick helped me to the living room couch and asked if my hands and feet were itching. I shook my head. It wasn't anaphylactic shock, but it was the worst asthma attack I ever remembered having.

"Get . . . my . . . adrenalin," I managed to say.

Meri rushed to the refrigerator to get the vial I kept there, while Vick hurried up the stairs to find a syringe. I had always hidden in a bathroom or a bedroom when I'd given myself injections in the past, but this time I knew I didn't have enough breath to move to a more private place. With shaking hands, I drew the adrenalin into the needle then pulled up the hem of my skirt and pushed the needle into my nylon-encased thigh.

Slumping back against the cushions, I tried to regulate my breathing by taking long inhalations instead of short gasps. I closed my eyes and concentrated on slowing my breathing pattern, knowing that the adrenalin would take effect within minutes. When my breathing became less labored and I felt the situation was under control, I opened my eyes. For the first time, I was acutely aware of my loved ones. Vick was sitting on the edge of the coffee table facing me and running his hands through his snow white hair. The girls were sitting together on the chair across the room, their brown eyes wide and horrified. They have never seen me give myself a shot before, and I could see the experience had been shocking to them.

"I'm sorry you had to see that," I said. Vick grasped my hand and squeezed it, and the girls ran over to hug me.

"Are you okay now, Momma?" Meri's voice shook and her eyes were brimming with tears.

I nodded and held both of my girls close. It had been a frightening attack, but it was over.

Vick cleared his throat and went over to the table. He began boxing up the stationery supplies. "I'll put this mess away. I don't think any of us are in the mood to stuff envelopes any more."

I lay back on the pillows of the rust-colored couch and the girls sat on the floor, still needing to be close to me, to touch me, to be sure their mother was all right.

"Does it hurt when you give yourself a shot?" asked Meri, her voice trembling. "I could never do that."

"I never thought I could either, honey, but I'm sure glad I learned how. I guess it stings a little bit, but by the time I need an injection, I'm so worried about my breathing that I don't notice the needle."

Kathy looked at me earnestly. "I want to learn how to give you a shot, Mom. Will you teach me, so that if you ever become unconscious I can do it for you?"

The thought appalled me, but I knew it would give my daughter comfort to feel she could help me if that need arose. "Yes, Trink, I'll show you how."

Abruptly Vick's shout interrupted me. "Oh, my God, look at this." He ran into the room and thrust the envelope box in front of my face.

There it was, on the label of the box.

"Premium Sulphite."

How had we ever missed it?

I sunk back into the pillow once again, overcome by the implication. I raised my eyes and looked at Vick.

"Do you suppose . . . ."

Our supposition was right. The next morning I called the paper mill from my office and discovered that, yes, the use of sulfiting agents was widespread in the paper industry. "It's less expensive than cotton rag," the mill's supervisor told me.

I thanked the man for the information and hung up, then sat with my head in my hands. If I believed in conspiracies, if I were paranoid, I'd feel certain that someone was out to get me.

In how many other ways would I accidentally confront sulfites? How many other ingenious uses for the chemical would I discover? Would something as innocent as licking an envelope kill me someday?

Suddenly I knew what I had to do. I couldn't control chance encounters with sulfites, but I could eliminate the known enemies. I'd take Dr. Stevens' advice. I'd continue to avoid sulfites in my diet and I'd move to a smog-free area.

I looked around my attractively paneled office and thought how much I'd miss it and all it represented. I'd worked so hard to get through school and to establish myself in a career I loved. Could I really just turn my back and walk away?

I knew I had no choice. I was only 36 years old, but my body was deteriorating with each breath of smog-filled air I took. I glanced at my office wall, and my eyes swept over the numerous plaques and scrolls I'd won for my writing and editing skills.

Yes, I'd miss all of this. But what good was a wall full of awards to a dead woman?

15

I raised my head from the oak desk and took a deep breath. I had no time for tears, no time for grief. I'd made my decision and now it was time to plan my departure. Pushing my chair away from the desk, I stood up and walked over to shut my office door. I looked guiltily at the stack of work I should be tackling, then pushed it aside. I felt like a short-timer already, but I had to start mapping out my escape.

A rush of emotion interfered with my logic. How could I take the girls away from their friends? How could I leave the man I loved? Tears began to sting my eyes, but I brushed them aside. I won't think about that now. I'll think about it tomorrow.

Oh, God, now I'm beginning to sound like Scarlett O'Hara.

I flipped through my desk calendar. The summer would be a good time to make a move. Kathy would be graduating from high school in June and would be leaving her friends behind anyway to live on campus at Cal Poly where she would begin majoring in Zoology. Meri was graduating from junior high and would be facing a new experience when she entered high school. I'd just have to find a way to convince her that facing that new experience in a new place would be exciting.

But what new place? I'd heard of a job opening in the Bay Area. Was San Francisco free of smog? Or how about Hawaii? Moving to the islands just might make leaving more bearable. Meri would love Maui.

That evening I broke the news to the girls. We were sitting around the dining room table, sharing the events of our days with each other as we did almost every night.

"We have to do a book report for Mr. Burke's class," Meri said. "What was that book you liked so much about that little boy and his hunting dogs?" she asked Kathy.

I watched the two of them discuss *Where the Red Fern Grows* and thought what pretty young women they had become. Kathy was so tall—five feet, eleven—and had a face and figure that were already turning the heads of men much older than she. Meri was a smaller-boned version of her older sister. In fact, many people thought they looked enough alike to be twins. They had identical "Colgate-bright" smiles, and each of them had a dimple in her chin.

"Dimple in the chin, where the devil goes in," I had always teased them. But there was nothing devilish about these two. They were beautiful, intelligent and compassionate individuals, and I not only loved them, I liked them.

"How was your day, Mom?" Both girls turned their attention to me.

"Well, it was quite a day. I've made a decision that is going to affect all of us."

I told them of my call to the paper mill, of my doctor's continual insistence that I move, of my resolve to do everything in my power to improve my health.

"I've decided that I have to leave Orange County and all this smog."

I plunged ahead, before either girl could respond.

"Kathy, you're going to be leaving anyway to begin a new life in college." I turned to my younger daughter. "And Meri, you and I will just have to be roommates somewhere else."

Both girls began to cry, and I felt tears begin to blind my eyes, too. I tried to keep my voice from shaking. "Kathy, with you I feel like a mother bird that has to encourage her baby to leave the nest and learn to fly."

My eyes met Meri's. "I know the thought of a move is scary for you, honey. You're probably wondering where we'll go, what school you'll attend and who your friends will be."

She nodded, wiping the wetness from her cheeks with a napkin. "I'm scared, too," I told her. "But wherever we go, we'll be together."

We all held hands, struggling with our emotions, all trying to be strong for each other.

"It's okay, Momma," Meri's voice broke. "You know I'd go anywhere if it means you can be well."

I smiled at my daughters. I had known they wouldn't disappoint me. They were beautiful on the inside, too.

Later that evening, Vick stopped by. He had been the master of ceremonies at a Press Club event, but I had known he would drop by on his way to the small apartment he called home in Anaheim.

Kathy and Meri were upstairs, honoring my wish to be alone with my dear friend. I wanted privacy, so I could tell him of the impending changes in my life.

He'd brought along a Presto-log and was busy preparing the fireplace as he regaled me with stories of his evening—who had been there, what had been said, funny scenarios that he thought I'd enjoy.

He finished his monologue just as the log caught fire, then turned to me, suddenly aware that he had been carrying on a one-sided conversation.

Joining me on the couch, he put his arm around me. "Hey, you're certainly quiet tonight."

I'd been rehearsing speeches in my mind for the last two hours, trying to find just the right words to tell Vick that I was leaving the area, leaving my job, leaving him. Now, however, I couldn't remember any of the tactful orations I'd practiced.

"I'm moving away," I blurted.

He sat sideways on the couch and looked at me. "What do you mean?"

Once again I chronicled the events of the day and my subsequent determination to fight the sulfites I could by living in a smog-free environment and paying strict attention to the foods I ate.

Vick was flabbergasted. "Where will you go?"

Fatigue swept over me, and I slouched into the corner of the couch. "I don't know yet."

"Well, I'll tell you one thing—you're not going alone."

Now it was my turn to ask him what he meant.

"I meant exactly what I said. Do you really think I'll let you leave without me?"

"Please, Vick, don't say something on the spur of the moment that you'll regret later. You've got your career to think of, your . . ."

He interrupted me with a kiss. "I love you. Wherever you and the kids go, I go, too."

"But . . ."

"Listen, I've changed careers three times, I can do it again."

He reached for me and pulled me into his arms, hiding his face in my hair. His voice was muffled, but I thrilled to his words. "I love you. I don't want to lose you."

Vick didn't return to his lonely apartment that night.

The next few weeks passed in a whirlwind of activity. I gave notice at work, put my condominium on the market and began making plans for a high school graduation, a junior high school promotion—and a wedding.

16

N*ow you will feel no rain, for each of you will be a shelter to the other. Now you will feel no cold, for each of you will be warmth to the other. Now there is no more lonliness, for each of you will be a companion to the other. Go now to your dwelling place to begin the days of your togetherness. May your days be long upon the earth, and may the wind always be at your backs."*

Surrounded by family and close friends, Vick and I leaned toward each other and shared our first kiss as husband and wife. A warm June breeze seemed to whisper its blessing as it softly rustled the leaves of the huge old tree under which we stood. We had decided to get married in the small, enclosed garden at Childrens Hospital, where Vick worked and where we had met six years before.

We smiled at each other and kissed again, before turning to accept the embraces and best wishes of our children, parents, sisters and other loved ones.

Happy shouts and applause suddenly broke the solemn spell, and we all looked up to see youngsters' faces leaning out of the window of the oncology ward, as the boys and girls tossed bird seed in lieu of rice over the garden below.

Vick caught the eye of one of his young friends, Gary Floyd, and waved.

"Hey, Vick," Gary yelled down in his raspy, adolescent voice, "Mrs. Knight is pretty."

Mrs. Knight! That was me. I was now Mrs. Vick Knight, Jr. It had all happened so fast. Had it only been three months before that I had made the decision that had changed the course of my life?

After a beautiful reception and an overnight honeymoon, the main item on our agenda was finding a place to live. I had called the Air Quality Management District for advice on smog-free areas in Southern California. The AQMD manager had been most helpful in researching the problem for me and suggested we explore the high desert area.

Vick and I spent two weekends looking at homes, visiting the Chambers of Commerce and investigating the high schools in communities such as Yucca Valley and Morongo. In the meantime, my new husband placed a call to the president of his professional organization, asking him to keep an eye open for positions in hospital fund-raising or public relations in desert areas.

One afternoon Vick called me at the office and said he'd just spoken with J.R. Nanetti, a photographer for an Orange County newspaper. J.R. and his family had moved to the Lake Elsinore area the year before and described their new hometown as hot and dry with clean air at least 90 percent of the time.

"Check the area out with your friends at the AQMD," Vick said. "If what J.R. says is true, we could live in that vicinity, and I could keep my job at CHOC—it's only 50 miles away."

It seemed too good to be true, but I placed a call to the air quality office and inquired about the Elsinore Valley. "We have no reports of any first stage smog alerts in that area," a woman told me.

I was surprised. I had believed Riverside County to be one of the worst areas for air pollution in California. However, air currents that made the Lake Elsinore region such a favorite for hot-air balloonists and hang glider enthusiasts also swept away the smog, I was told.

The next weekend we investigated Lake Elsinore and found it to be a sleepy rural town, surrounding a large lake that reflected the towering mountains above it. We were even more captivated by the private community of Canyon Lake, just three miles east. The beautiful resort-like area had so many amenities—a golf course, a lake, beaches and parks, tennis courts, an equestrian center, a lodge and a swimming pool.

Vick and I stood under a giant allepo pine on the upper deck of the country club there and watched the water skiers zipping by on the lake. Turning, we gazed toward the snow-capped peaks above San Bernardino, then up at the royal blue sky, so unlike the murky gray-brown outdoor ceiling we were accustomed to in Orange County.

I squeezed Vick's hand. "This is the place."

Now the serious house-hunting began. Even on the days that Vick could not join us because of other commitments, Meri and I continued the search. My younger daughter was equally as enthused about the area and, as a real water lover, the idea of living on a lake was a dream come true.

We knew the house was made for us the minute we saw it. Overlooking the sixteenth fairway, the place had three levels and was built on a gently sloping cliff. The upper two stories included sun porches across the back offering an almost pastoral view. I could picture us sitting there sipping lemonade or mint juleps—anything but wine—and watching the sun go down. Within three days, Meri, Kathy, Vick and I had visited the house four times, and by the end of the week, it was ours.

Relocating two households of furniture and three carloads of wedding and graduation gifts 50 miles in a U-Haul truck would not be anyone's idea of fun. A major move is traumatic under the best of circumstances—and it was especially so for the girls, who were leaving the area they'd lived in for almost all their lives. Even Vick was more solemn than usual, and he urged us all to sit down for a non-hurried breakfast of donuts and milk before we began. Afterwards we all looked at each other and held hands.

Knowing that tempers operated on a short fuse under such stressful conditions, Vick gave us a little pep talk. "Let's hope we're as good friends by tonight as we are right now," he concluded.

We were—and by nightfall we were even semi-organized. The 3100 square-foot house swallowed our furniture, and the next morning we sat on the floor of the sunporch making a list of items we needed, then assigned a priority to them.

"I think we need a hot tub," Kathy said, trying to keep a straight face.

Meri quickly jumped into the spirit of things. "No, what we need first is a dog."

Vick cleared his throat. Standing up and stretching to take advantage of his 65 inches of height, he tried to affect an authoritarian demeanor.

"I'm the man of the house now, and I say our first order of business is a fence around the backyard."

The girls and I laughed. "A fence?" we said in unison. The rolling hills and openess of this beautiful community had attracted us to the area. Who needed a fence?

"We definitely need a fence to keep the rabbits away from the vineyard I'm going to plant."

I stood up and pushed Vick's arm playfully. "You sit down." I faced my family and began counting off the items I thought we needed more than a spa, a puppy or a bunch of grapevines.

"You're sitting on the floor right now because we don't have any patio furniture," I said. "We slept on a couch in the den last night because there's no furniture in the master bedroom. Our living room is bare, the kitchen needs . . ."

Vick and the girls jumped up. Vick put his hands over my mouth and Kathy and Meri began to tickle me. "Okay, okay, you win," they all said.

But, I didn't.

On the first Saturday in our new home, I had to return to the office in Orange County to gather my personal belongings and to organize the files for the next corporate editor. Leaving had been even more painful than I had anticipated, and my last week had been spent saying goodbye to friends and being treated to surprise luncheons. Consequently I had not accomplished the cleanup tasks I had hoped to, so I made arrangements with security to enter the building over the weekend.

It was six hours later that, chores accomplished, I arrived back home. Vick ran out to the garage to meet me, helped me add several more boxes to the stacks of cartons still waiting to be unpacked, then looked at me with a sheepish grin.

"I have something to show you, sweetie," he said leading me by the hand. "Now, if you don't like it, I've got the man's word that he'll take it back."

What in the world? I allowed Vick to guide me down the stairs and around the corner with my eyes closed.

"Surprise."

My eyes flew open, and there in the middle of the back room was a pool table—next to last on our list of priorities.

"Isn't it great? I had the man use rust-colored felt so that it would match the carpeting."

Still in shock, I watched my husband hurry around the table, racking balls and pointing out the wonderful features of his new toy.

"The man had to assemble it right here on the premises. There was no way he could have gotten it down the stairs and through the door otherwise. But he promised to take it back if you don't like it."

I still hadn't said a word. Vick walked over to me and nuzzled my neck. "May I keep it, Mommy? Please?"

I had to smile. Why fight it?

"You can keep it on one condition," I said, laughing. "You have to put a mattress on it every night so that we can use it as a bed until we can afford a bedroom set."

Within a month we were settled in our new environment and happily establishing a new routine. I took advantage of the warm, crystal clear days by spending as much time as possible with the girls. Kathy would be leaving for college in the fall—and who knew when we'd be able to share a summer together again. It was important to me to establish Canyon Lake as *home* in her mind—and I only had two months in which to do so. I took special pains to help her decorate the small bedroom overlooking the golf course so that she would consider it *hers*.

We spent long, lazy days on the beach, fine-tuning our tans and enjoying each other's company. My job had kept me so busy and involved that I'd forgotten how much I missed having leisure time to spend with my daughters. Vick bought us a three-man rubber boat and we paddled along the lake, getting acquainted with the coves and waterways of our new community.

Soon, however, it was time to turn the pages of the calendar. September had arrived and, with it, the new school year. With a lump in my throat I helped Kathy move into her ten-by-ten dorm room and left her, feeling as if I'd left a part of my heart.

Meri started school within a week of her sister, and on her first day of classes, I hugged her goodbye, watched her walk to the school bus stop, then kissed Vick as he headed for Orange County and his job there.

I closed the door and felt very alone.

I walked slowly through my new home, fluffing a pillow on the couch here and rearranging a knick-knack there before sitting down on the sunporch and staring at the golfers moving around the fairway in their colorful little golfcarts.

I felt almost as if I'd entered a time capsule and was reliving another part of my life. Granted I had new scenery—and even a new name, but here I was again, exiling myself from "the real world."

Of course this time my eyes were wide open and I knew what I was doing and why. However, the end result suddenly seemed the same. I was at home alone while the world was passing me by.

I got up and went inside, walking into the upstairs office, which we had furnished with a large desk, a typewriter and a reference library. It was here that I hoped to someday establish a freelance business.

The phone rang, making me jump as the loud jangle reverberated on all four extensions in the empty barn of a house.

"Hello Carolyn. Dr. Stevens here. I thought you'd like to know that we've just documented another woman who is allergic to sulfiting agents."

"You have?" Just as I had suspected. I wasn't alone in the world after all. "I'd love to talk to her."

"I was hoping you'd say that. With your permission I'd like to give Jo Valone your phone number so that she can gain from your experience and your insight into the problem."

"Oh, yes, please feel free to do that."

"You know, Carolyn, we're considering your discovery a medical breakthrough," my doctor continued. "We believe there are at least 500,000 other asthmatics in the United States alone who are sulfite sensitive—and maybe as many as a million."

I was stunned. I sat dumbly, waiting for Dr. Stevens to continue.

"You are a very special person, my friend. Thousands of others could have had the same clues you did and never would have put two and two together."

My cheeks burned, and I swallowed hard. "Dr. Stevens, I think you're exaggerating. You deserve *my* thanks. You don't know how much I appreciate having a doctor who listens and who encourages patients to take an active role in their health care."

"Well then, we have a mutual admiration society," said my doctor. "And, by the way, we have a new nickname for you here at the Clinic. We've begun calling you the Queen Bee of Metabisulfites."

We laughed, then exchanged goodbyes and hung up.

Suddenly the house didn't seem so lonely anymore. I felt more motivated than I ever had in my life, and I looked around my little office with new eyes.

From here I'd begin a one-woman battle against sulfites. I'd research the subject and share what I'd learn with the world. Dr. Stevens had said there might be as many as a million others out there somewhere as afraid and bewildered as I'd been for so many years.

I felt a kinship with Jo Valone and those unknown thousands of others and made a silent vow. I'd carry the banner for all of us.

My crusade had begun.

17

My new resolve had to be postponed almost before it began. Perhaps Meri brought a flu bug home from school, or Vick a virus from the office. Maybe I had fallen victim to food poisoning. Whatever the reason, *I was sick.* For three days, I lay in bed unable to move. I could keep nothing on my stomach and, during my more lucid moments, I was concerned that I was losing my asthma medications along with the foods my family kept encouraging me to try.

On the fourth day of my dreadful malady, I opened my eyes and felt as if I might live after all. Supported by wobbly legs, I joined Vick and Meri in the family room.

My daughter rushed to my side to help me to the couch. "Mom are you sure you should be up? Would you like me to fix you something to eat?"

My stomach turned at the thought. "No thanks, honey. Maybe just a cup of tea, please."

Vick joined me on the couch. "Are you breathing okay? Have you been able to take your pills today?"

"This last dose was the first I've been able to keep down in more than three days," I replied. "The funny thing is, though, that I haven't had any asthma symptoms at all, despite the lack of medication."

The next morning I felt much stronger and was able to eat a light breakfast. After seeing Vick and Meri off, I thought about the events of the last few days. I'd been completely relieved of any breathing problems and, thinking back, I recalled that, on the rare occasions in my life that I had fasted, I had enjoyed asthma-free days, also.

Hmm, fasting. Why would my asthma be so much better on an empty stomach?

Figuratively putting on my detective's cap once more, I wondered if part of my problem could be caused by food allergies. I called Dr. Stevens and made an appointment to discuss my hypothesis with him.

As usual the good doctor listened to my reasoning with an open mind as I sat in his Clinic office and listed my reasons for believing I might be allergic to foods.

I opened my purse and pulled out an ad I'd clipped from the newspaper the Sunday before. Since my humiliation over mentioning urine injections to Dr. Rice so long ago, I had ignored accounts of miracle cures. However, a large advertisement discussing food allergies had caught my eye because of its testimonials from all kinds of people—including Merv Griffin. One asthmatic woman who had previously been on a breathing machine several times a day had been dramatically helped by what was being termed cytotoxic examination.

I held out the ad to my doctor. "Do you think we could use this method to discover whether or not I'm allergic to foods?"

Dr. Stevens politely looked at the ad. Cytotoxic testing involved exposing a person's blood to over 200 common foods and additives. If the person's white cells exploded upon contact with a substance, allergy was indicated. It sounded like an exciting new procedure to me. Normal allergy testing involved being "scratched" with various allergens and waiting to see whether or not the skin reacted by producing ugly red weals. However, the accuracy of this type of testing with foodstuffs was only successful 20 percent of the time, I'd been told. On the other hand, cytotoxic testing involved drawing a small vial of blood—and it was being touted as being accurate 80 to 90 percent of the time.

I tried to read Dr. Stevens face as he scanned the wordy advertisement. Frown lines gathered on his forehead and his eyes narrowed behind his aviator glasses.

"I know the method of advertising this new testing method is rather sensationalized," I said, trying to let him know that I realized cytotoxic testing was not an accepted medical procedure. Neither was advertising for that matter.

"We have to take some of their claims with a grain of salt," I continued. "After all they say they can cure everything from pimples and obesity to arthritis and ulcers."

I laughed and then became more serious. "Dr. Stevens, I'm willing to explore even the newest and more unorthodox means to help me get well. I've left my job and have moved to a supposedly smog-free area, but I'm still plagued with this damned disease, so something else *must* be adding to it."

I warmed to my subject. "We live in a plastic, synthetic world today. Not all allergies fall into the neat categories that doctors have used for years. Not everybody is going to be allergic to the old standbys like dog dander, grasses, molds or house dust. At least the lab in this advertisement is offering to admit that other allergens exist—and they've developed a new procedure to test them."

"Carolyn, I agree that the medical profession must be willing to accept more modern and unconventional answers to old problems as they come along. Since your discovery of sulfite-sensitivity, I've been even more convinced of that than ever. But, I consider those conducting cytotoxic examinations nothing but quacks."

I sat back in my chair, surprised at my physician's strong reaction.

"First of all, a white blood cell lives only four hours, and when a blood sample is drawn, there is no way to determine how old these cells are. So, if a cell explodes when you douse it with milk or wheat extract or some food additive, did it self-destruct because of allergy or because of old age?"

I shook my head and shrugged my shoulders, ashamed that I had been willing again to believe an advertisement rather than a trusted physician and friend. If cytotoxic testing had been legitimate, Dr. Stevens would have been among the first to sing its praises and to incorporate its procedures.

"If you want to test yourself for food allergy, try this," He handed me a copy of an elimination diet.

During the 1940's, an allergist had found that patients suffering from chronic bronchitis and asthma often improved dramatically by adhering to his strict food plan.

"I haven't found that to be the case with my own patients," said Dr. Stevens, "but perhaps nobody has really given the diet a fair chance."

I could understand why! Instead of listing foods one should avoid, the diet consisted of a sparse list of foods one could eat:

Tapioca
White Potato
Soy Bean Potato Bread
Lima Bean Potato Bread
Soy Bean Milk
Lamb
Chicken (no hens)
Bacon (Swift or Dubuque)
Liver (lamb, beef)
Artichoke
Asparagus
Beets
Carrots
Chard
Garbanzos
Lettuce
Lima Beans
Peas
Spinach
Squash
String Beans
Tomatoes
Apricots
Grapefruit
Lemons
Peaches
Prunes
Pears
Pineapple
C&H Sugar
Brown Sugar
Molasses
Salt
Sesame Oil
Soy Bean Oil
Willow Run Margarine
Knox's Gelatin
Maple Syrup, made with Cane Sugar
White Vinegar
Vanilla Extract
Lemon Extract
Corn-Free Baking Powder
Baking Soda
Cream of Tartar
Rum (Puerto Rican and Jamaican)
Club Soda

"If you want to give this diet a try, stay on it for three weeks," my doctor said. "After that you can begin adding foods one at a time every five days."

Dr. Stevens threw me a teasing look, as if he thought I was searching for an excuse not to try the diet.

"I know what you're thinking, Doc, but you're wrong. I'll not only start your diet, I'll stick to it religiously. Who knows, maybe it will help me solve this mystery I call my life."

18

My stomach rumbling, I sat the the breakfast bar in the kitchen and, for the fourth time that day, scanned the diet. It had been in my hands almost constantly for the past two weeks as I carried it around trying to think of some appetizing way to prepare the meager list of foods. Vick and Meri had begun to tease me about my preoccupation with food and my continual reading of the booklet.

"You should have that thing memorized by now," Vick kept commenting.

"I do. I do," I assured him. "I'm just looking for loopholes."

The diet was even scantier now that I had modified it for my sulfite sensitivity. Despite the fact that it allowed canned fruits and vegetables, I knew they were preserved with sulfites, so I eliminated all but the ones that were in season and available at the fresh produce section of the market. I also crossed off the vinegar, knowing that, if wine contained SO_2, vinegar would too. I couldn't find either brand of bacon that the diet allowed (manufactured by companies that did not cure the meat in corn syrup) so that left it out—and how in the world do you find out if the chicken you're buying is male or female? I decided not to take a chance and drew a line through chicken, also.

My taste buds made further modifications. No matter how hard I tried, I just couldn't swallow soy bean or lima bean potato bread. Yuck. Soy bean milk tasted like wallpaper paste. I'd never developed a liking for liver or sweet potatoes and I couldn't figure out what to do with the tapioca, the molasses, the syrup, the extracts, the baking soda and powder, the gelatin or the cream of tartar.

My meals were beginning to all resemble one another: a hamburger patty, a baked potato and a sliced tomato or salad with fresh fruit for dessert—breakfast, lunch and dinner.

"Thank God for the rum," I joked to Vick. "It gives me a brighter outlook on life."

I was losing weight fast—not good for a woman who already was an Olive Oyl look-alike. But I was better. In fact, my asthma had improved dramatically from the first day of dieting.

To emphasize the point I took out my small peak flow meter and blew heartily into its mouthpiece to measure the air I could expend in one breath. I looked at the needle. Yes, I'd been able to push it past 400 again. In the past the best I could "blow" on *good* days was 300.

The diet was definitely having a profound effect, so some food I'd been eating in the past must have really exacerbated my condition. Without it to trigger an allergic response, I'd been able to reduce my cortisone dosages to 10 mg per day, down from frequent highs of 25, 30 and even 40 mg per day.

But what food could it be? What did I eat enough of each and every day to keep my asthma flaring continuously?

Or was it food at all?

Maybe it was a food additive, an artificial color, another preservative.

Or maybe the use of sulfiting agents was even more widespread than I'd thought.

One thing was certain—every bite that had gone into my mouth in the past fourteen days had been fresh, so I ingested no SO_2.

I picked up the phone and called Kathy at her dorm at Cal Poly. I knew the college offered a food technology degree, so I prevailed on my older daughter for help.

"Honey, I know your classes are really keeping you busy, but would you stop by the school library before you come home this weekend and see if there are any books available on sulfur dioxide or the use of sulfiting agents in foods?"

She arrived home Saturday morning with a roommate, a hamper full of dirty laundry, a stack of homework to be completed before Monday—and a book by Dr. Louis Schroeter, published by Pergamon Press, entitled *Sulfur Dioxide: Applications in Foods, Beverages and Pharmaceuticals.*

I held the volume much like a preacher would hold a Bible. "I can't believe there's such a book," I told her. "From the title, it sounds as if it were written for my benefit."

I spent the entire weekend sitting at my desk poring over the very technical text. I was not an uneducated person, but science had never been my strong point. I struggled with the chemical formulas and analytical explanations, but most of the information was over my head.

Midway through the book, however, Dr. Schroeter began writing in a language I could understand.

" . . . sulfur dioxide is one of the most common food and beverage preservatives."

" . . . harmless in the amounts normally employed."

"The safety of sufites . . . is generally conceded even by those critical of the excessive use of food additives and preservatives."

The author then began listing foods that benefited from the use of this widely used additive. Not only was sulfur dioxide used in fruits and vegetables, as I'd been told, it was also used in sugar to keep it from fermenting, in flour to protect it from microorganisms, in dried milk, garlic powder, tapioca, corn starch . . .

I couldn't control my shock any longer. "I can't believe this," I screamed at the top of my lungs.

My family came running. "What's wrong?"

"Listen to this." I continued to read Dr. Schroeter's list of foods that used the anti-oxident that was my own personal adversary.

"Sulfites are everywhere," I said. "They're in soups, iodized salt, bread and pastry and pizza doughs, beer, cognac, syrups, jams, jellies, juices, carbonated drinks . . . "

My voice broke. "They're even added to citric and ascorbic acids. I'd always felt safe eating foods preserved with those."

I closed the book. "No wonder I've been sick all these years—there's no way to avoid this stuff without starving to death. You might as well order my coffin right now."

My family didn't know what to say or how to comfort me. They'd seen me angry about my asthma. They'd seen me depressed. But they'd never heard such desperation in my voice before. They'd never heard me give up.

I pushed past their outstretched arms, oblivious to their words of caring, and hurried down the stairs and into my bedroom. I closed the door behind me, crawled under the covers of the king-sized bed and assumed a fetal position. Why try to fight this invasive enemy?

It wasn't long before I felt another body cradling mine, spoon fashion. Vick hugged me but offered support only through his presence, allowing my misery to run its course in silence. Despite the early hour, I fell asleep, soothed by the strength of his embrace.

I awakened an hour later, still encircled by my husband—and still morose. Vick, however, had experienced enough pessimism.

"Look on the bright side," he insisted. "Now you have an even better idea of what to fight—and you know it works. You've been feeling really terrific on this new diet."

He was right, of course. My research was uncovering information that could keep me living a much more healthy—and therefore a much more normal—life.

But I still wasn't smiling.

"God, Vick. I don't know if I can stand to eat hamburger patties and baked potatoes every day for the rest of my life."

My husband kissed my cheek and grinned. "I'm sure you'll find other foods you can eat."

He seemed relieved that I was only acting depressed now—anything was better than suicidal.

Suddenly I raised my voice. "Damn it, Vick. How do the manufacturers get away with using this . . . this *venom* in our food? It never appears on labels. No one's even heard of the stuff."

I continued shouting. "I found out about sulfiting agents strictly by accident—and now I discover that they're the most common preservatives used today.

"It's wrong. It's criminal. I can't believe they adulterate our food with toxic chemicals without our knowledge. They're not going to get away with this."

Vick began to applaud and the girls, who had been worriedly camped outside the bedroom, threw open the door and cheered.

"Hooray. Your mother's on the warpath again."

"All right, Momma."

"Go for it."

Evidently, my family felt that giving up was verboten, being depressed was so-so, being upset was okay—but being enraged was terrific.

19

I barely slept that night. Instead I listened to the sounds of the coyotes and owls echoing from the foothills surrounding our home and mapped my course for the future. I really didn't know just how to proceed, but decided to start with a phone call to Dr. Schroeter who, through his text, had opened my eyes to the momentous task I now faced.

Restless from tossing all night, yet surprisingly alert despite my lack of sleep, I sneaked out of bed at 5 a.m., tiptoeing so that I wouldn't awaken my still snoring husband.

I crept into my office, turned on the light and looked at the title page of the sulfur dioxide book. Dr. Schroeter had been employed by the Upjohn Company in 1966 when the book have been published. Was he still there 16 years later? Was the information still valid? Had it been updated?

I looked at the clock. It was only 5:15. With the time difference it would be 8:15 on the East Coast. I picked up the phone and asked the operator for the number of the pharmaceutical firm in Kalamazoo, Michigan, then dialed.

Yes, Dr. Schroeter was still with the company, I was told. He was now vice-president and general manager of the domestic pharmaceutical division. Within minutes I was speaking to perhaps the most knowledgeable person in the United States, if not the world, on the subject of sulfur dioxide.

"Dr. Schroeter, my name is Carolyn Knight, and I'm calling you from California because of a life-threatening allergy to sulfur dioxide."

The kind executive listened respectfully as I recounted the past years of my life and the mysterious illness that I'd just recently begun to understand. He was astounded that a chemical he had believed innocuous could have caused my problem, and he interjected words of surprise as our conversation continued.

Perhaps he expected me to compain about his study or to become angry about his conclusions that the chemical was a safe and effective preservative. But what purpose would that serve now? Instead I told him how much his book had helped me in solving the riddle I called asthma.

His research into $S0_2$ had ended shortly after his book was published, he told me, although he believed the work was still considered the definitive volume on the subject.

"The chapters in the book dealing with food and beverage applications were quite complete through 1965," he said. "But in science and technology that is a long, long time. Most likely the food technology professors at the University of California at Davis could provide you with more recent studies."

We talked a few more minutes, and Dr. Schroeter promised to send me his latest available copy of the book since it was no longer in print.

"I'm so pleased the information in my book has helped you with your health problems," he said as he hung up.

I closed my eyes and sighed, finally feeling tired from the strain of the long night. Yes, you've been a great help, Dr. Schroeter, but how I wish I'd had this information when I first got sick. I could have controlled my asthma through diet. Instead I had relied all these years on strong medications and was now dealing with the extreme side effects of some of them.

I was completely dependent on cortisone now, my own adrenal gland no longer supplied my body with the natural hormone but instead counted on the little white pills of prednisolone to do their work each morning.

My last trip to the ophthalmologist had confirmed my greatest fear—my eyes were beginning to cloud even more with the growth of cortisone-induced cataracts and, before too many years passed, I would face surgery to correct them. In addition, my joints were becoming increasingly affected by the powerful drug and, like an arthritic, I experienced great pain in my hips and knees if I did much walking.

And why was this happening? Why was my 38-year-old body falling apart like one twice its age? Because for years I'd been poisoned with almost every bite of food I'd eaten. I had to do something about this problem. I just had to.

I spent the next two weeks getting up early so that I could make long distance calls to food manufacturers and government agencies back east while taking advantage of the lower telephone rates. I contacted quality control managers at flour mills, at sugar refineries and at cooking oil manufacturers, among others, attempting to add sulfite-free staples to the foods I could safely consume.

A call to one natural food company seemed almost too good to be true.

"Our products are natural, which means nothing is removed or added," I was told by the director of consumer concerns.

However, a trip to a nearby health food store and a perusal of the company's labels sent me back to the phone to contact the executive again.

"Ma'am, your labels list the use of white flour and hydrogenated oil," I confronted her. "How can you call those products natural?"

"Well, white flour is an exception to the statement that nothing is removed," she admitted. "But we consider white flour a natural product."

I was stunned. According to Schroeter's book, white flour was treated with sulfur dioxide gas during processing.

"Your company's claims are untrue," I said into the receiver, trying to sound businesslike instead of emotional. "People like me, with life-threatening allergies, could become very ill by believing your advertising. Some of us might even die."

"Look, " she replied, "if you take the term *natural* verbatim to mean that the product is unadulterated in any way, that's a misconception."

I couldn't believe my ears. *I* was operating under a misconception because I believed her company's definition of natural? I hung up abruptly, grabbed my car keys and hurried to the grocery store with paper, a pen and a purpose.

I walked up and down aisle after aisle, picking up one "natural" product after another and reading more than 75 labels of foods touting "no preservatives added."

Natural soybean margarine? How could any margarine be natural when, by its very definition, it was imitation butter? What did Anheuser-Busch mean by Natural Light Beer? Beer contained sulfites and who knew what else. A "natural" bread contained mono- and dimonia-sulfates. A "natural" cheese contained food coloring. A "natural" yogurt contained powdered milk—which according to Dr. Schroeter contained sulfites. A "natural" soup mix contained hydrolized plant protein. What in the world was that? A "natural" flavored snack was made with monosodium glutamate. A "natural" juice apple pie contained artifical color and flavoring, mono- and dyglycerides and, guess what else? An anti-oxident. I'd be willing to bet it was sulfite.

The list went on.

My visual shopping spree complete, I hurried back home and placed a call to the Food and Drug Administration in Washington, D.C. Just as I'd begun to believe, the FDA, which regulates labeling, had never attempted to define the term "natural."

"We've taken no position on the use of the terms 'organic,' 'natural' or 'health' in regards to foods," the officer told me. "The only way to assure that a product labeled as 'organically grown' is truthfully labeled would be to keep watch over the product from planting to harvesting to sales, and to check soil and water reports. Such a program would be prohibitively expensive."

The Federal Trade Commission, which has jurisdiction over advertising had tried, I was told, not only to define "natural" but to regulate its use. However, the commission had run into one roadblock after another because the Reagan administration opposes any increase in regulation.

I hung up, realizing that the only thing for certain about health foods was that they cost more than conventional foods. It looked as if I were on my own. I would have to be totally responsible for every morsel of food I put into my mouth.

"Finding foods I can eat is beginning to be a full time job," I told Vick that night.

I did have some luck. I began ordering wheat from a mill in Texas, whose quality control manager assured me that their product was grown on the premises and wasn't sprayed in the field or in the processing with SO_2. I found a brand of cooking oil I could use, and although I was unable to locate any unsulfited sugar, I found that raw honey could be substituted quite satisfactorily in most recipes. And to think I used to laugh at health food nuts. Here I was becoming the Adele Davis of sulfites.

Each day my post office box seemed to contain more information to add to my growing research into the sulfite problem. The University of California at Davis sent me a status summary by the Institute of Food Technologists Expert Panel on Food Safety and Nutrition. Published in 1975, the report attempted to define how much sulfite per pound of body weight was safe for human consumption.

My hands shook as I read the report and I resisted the urge to crumple the paper and throw it into the wastepaper basket. What good was it to determine that the acceptable daily intake of SO_2 for a 155-pound person was 50 mg per day when foods were not labeled so that people like me could calculate how much of the chemical they were ingesting? A person drinking a half liter of wine could be ingesting 100 mg or more, I knew, and with the consumption of canned and processed foods rising each year. Data in the status summary indicated that the amount of SO_2 consumed per capita each day could reach 600 mg. I had reacted to 20 mg at the Clinic and had gone into anaphylactic shock at 50 mg.

My frustration grew. My asthmatic condition had improved tremendously, thanks to the information I'd found buried in scientific literature and to the dozens of phone calls I'd made. I did share my research with Jo Valone and the handful of others who had been diagnosed as sulfite-sensitive at Scripps. But what about the estimated one million others out there someplace who were living in danger because they did not have the facts I did?

What could I do to share my research with others? I was a writer—perhaps I should detail my discovery in a feature article and send it to some of the more popular national magazines, those that would reach the most readers.

"Carolyn, unfortunately, that's just not the way to go about it," Dr. Stevens told me as I sat in his office and discussed the issue. "Doctors just don't put much stock in the opinions of patients who come to them and tell them they think they have a disease they just read about in the *Reader's Digest.*"

"Well, I've got to do something. What do you suggest?"

Dr. Stevens sat back and studied me for a moment. "My associates and I have been bringing your case up at every doctors' conference we attend. We've seen light bulbs turn on all over the audience as other allergists begin frantically taking notes when we tell them about your experience with sulfites. The word *is* getting out—but slowly."

"And, in the meantime, I'm sure people are dying out there," I said, my voice choking. "Please think about it, Dr. Stevens, and let me know if there is anything I can do."

I walked to the parking lot and got into my car, feeling strangely despondent. I had just had a fantastic check-up. At one point in my life I would have been exhilarated by that fact and by the results of the research I was conducting. My health had improved dramatically. But I felt no such euphoria. Saving myself wasn't good enough. I wanted to save the one million others too.

20

Fire and brimstone.

I had heard the phrase so often in my church-going days when the preacher associated it with the devil, hell and all that was evil—and now here they were, the same words and fears confronting me again.

Brimstone.

The word popped off the page as I sat studying one of the textbooks I had checked out at the university library. Sulfur, I read, comes from the Latin word for brimstone, or burning. High priests thousands of years ago used sulfur in religious ceremonies, when the blue, pungent flame coming from the yellow rock helped the clergy create the belief that hell was fueled by brimstone.

That belief still had validity for me, I decided, as I continued to read.

I was attempting to broaden my research to include sources of sulfur dioxide in the environment, and now I was certain that, if ingesting the chemical didn't kill me, inhaling it would.

My own personal nemesis has many uses in the modern world, I was finding, and has had since 3000 B.C. when man first discovered it. The United States has the dubious honor of being the leading sulfur producer in the world, and one book I consulted said that more than 50 million tons of sulfur are produced and released into our environment annually, with an additional 60 million tons of man-made SO_2 emissions given off each year.

Sulfur dioxide is used in the paper, petroleum, fertilizer, steel, copper and uranium-ore industries. It is used in the manufacture of bleaching and anti-chlorinating agents . . . in the treatment of water supplies . . . in boiler waters and in cleaning wells . . . in the production of glass, paints, explosives and detergents. It is used in the tanning of leather . . . in the processing of textiles . . . in the vulcanizing of rubber.

The dangerous chemical is discharged from the burning of bituminous coal . . . from electric power generating plants . . . from smelters, petroleum refineries, coking operations. It is emitted from the combustion of gasoline, kerosene . . .

It is everywhere. I had to be inhaling SO_2 with every breath I took.

I turned again to the book. Tall stacks, used to send the chemical far into the upper atmosphere actually spread the emissions over a much larger area, I read—and the sulfur dioxide finds its way to earth again in the form of acid rain.

Acid rain! I'd heard so much about that recently. But I didn't know the acid they were talking about was composed of SO_2. No wonder I was so often sick when it rained.

I read on. Ecologist Dr. Anne LaBastille, consultant to the Smithsonian Institution and author of many scientific books, was quoted as blaming acid rain for many deaths. "The possibility exists that there could be 50,000 deaths related to acid rain," she said, "the majority from respiratory and cardiac illnesses."

It got worse.

Acid fog was another enemy. According to *Science Magazine*, the deadly fog was more corrosive and dangerous than acid rain. Researchers from Cal Tech now believe that London's five-day killer fog of 1952 that caused 12,000 deaths from bronchitis and heart disease was an example of acid fog, the article reported.

The joke's on me, I thought with a macabre sense of humor. I'd uprooted my family to avoid the smog of the city. But how does a person move away from acid fog or rain? I was sure that sulfur dioxide emissions from vehicles, refineries and industries all over Southern California found their way over the hills and into the valleys of Canyon Lake in those forms.

Was there no way to beat it? Was I allergic to the modern, industrialized world?

Surely this problem was too big for me to tackle by myself. All of a sudden my shoulders sagged, and I was overwhelmed by the crusade I had undertaken. It would take a miracle for one little person to make any headway in this battle—and by now I knew that miracles just didn't exist.

Enter Michael Jacobson, miracle worker.

I went to my post office box the following week and tore open an envelope from my doctors at the Clinic. In it was a photocopy of a letter addressed to Dr. Stevens from the executive director of the Center for Science in the Public Interest. With headquarters in Washington, D.C., Mike Jacobson's consumer advocacy group wanted to tackle the issue of sulfiting agents in foods by petitioning the FDA.

"Dr. Jacobson asked me to alert our SO_2-sensitive patients to his campaign," a note from my physician read. He went on to explain that Jacobson was researching a book he had titled *Chemicals in Your Booze* when he became aware of the use of sulfiting agents in wine. That had led him to the Clinic—and to me.

Goose bumps tingled up and down my arms. This just might be the breakthrough I needed.

I rushed back to my house and, too impatient to write, phoned Dr. Jacobson the minute I reached my office.

"Mrs. Knight, I'm glad you called," he said. "Your doctor indicated you might be willing to sign a petition we're bringing before the FDA. We want to pressure the agency to greatly curtail or ban the use of these dangerous chemicals in foods."

"You're an answer to my prayers, Dr. Jacobson. I was beginning to feel like the proverbial little voice crying out in the wilderness. I can't believe your organization is willing to help. But isn't there something I can do besides add my name to a petition?"

"As a matter of fact, there is. I understand you're a writer. Would you be willing to provide us with a statement on how sulfiting agents have affected your life? I'd like to attach it to a news release we're sending out."

I swiveled back and forth in my chair. "Writing a book would be easier, I joked. "But I'll see what I can do."

I gave him permission to use my name in his action against the government agency, promised him my written statement would be in the morning's mail and closed the conversation with my new collaborator on a first name basis.

Rolling a piece of paper into my typewriter, I stared at the blank sheet for several minutes. How could I possibly summarize the agony of my asthma-inflicted years in one or two paragraphs? My quip to Mike about a book held more truth than fiction. I could write chapters on the subject.

Suddenly, however, my fingers began to fly and, within 15 minutes I had prepared a statement for release.

> *Sulfiting agents, considered harmless preservatives by the federal government and godsends by the food industry, have had a monumental impact on my life. Although I have attempted to avoid antioxidants, they are so common in the air we breath and the meals we eat, that I have had nine life-threatening bouts with anaphylactic shock and have endured the daily heartache of chronic asthma for more than 10 years. Besides living with the day to day shortness of breath which deprives me of leading a normally active life, I live with the fear that I will accidentally encounter the substance that can, within 10 minutes, snuff out my life if I do not receive immediate help.*
>
> *I am on daily cortisone therapy, which in itself is dangerous to my health, and take myriad other medications to keep my airways open. I eat NO processed, frozen or prepared foods, which limits my diet immensely. I carry adrenalin with me at all times, ready to inject myself when respiratory arrest threatens. In more far-reaching consequences of the GRAS chemical, I have uprooted my family to settle in an area with lesser concentrations of smog and have had to take leave from the career I had worked toward for so many years.*

My statement was released and picked up by United Press International accompanying the article prepared by Jacobson and his staff. Newspaper throughout the United States were suddenly alerting readers to the dangers of sulfites.

> *WASHINGTON—A widely used food preservative that has been approved by the Food and Drug Administration could bring some people, particularly asthma sufferers, to "the brink of death" a consumer group charged yesterday.*
>
> *Michael Jacobson, executive director of the Center for Science in the Public Interest, accused the FDA of being "asleep again" and of making a "terribly poor" review of the safety of sodium bisulfite and related chemicals before approving their use a food perservatives.*
>
> *At a news conference at the Capital, Jacobson said the center is petitioning the FDA "to ban or severely curtail" the use of sodium bisulfite, potassium metabisulfite and sulfur dioxide for the preservation of foods.*
>
> *"It makes no sense to allow in our food supply a chemical that brings people to the brink of death," he said.*
>
> *Jacobson said studies by doctors at the Scripps Clinic and Research Foundation in La Jolla, California, proved that many people—particularly asthmatics—are sensitive to sulfiting agents.*
>
> *Clinic doctors, in a statement released by Jacobson, said bisulfite caused faintness, shortness of breath, severe wheezing and even loss of consciousness in some of their patients. He estimated that 400,000 to one million asthmatics are "endangered" by sulfiting agents and "an unknown number" of other people also are affected by the chemicals.*
>
> *Jacobson said the food industry uses tens of millions of pounds of sulfites every year to preserve packaged foods, shrimp and other shellfish, most wines and beer.*
>
> *He said an FDA decision to ban or restrict the use of sulfites in food should be "quick and easy," because safer substitutes are available. But he said the center would appeal to the courts if the FDA does not act within "a reasonable" time—from six months to a year.*
>
> *A spokesman for the FDA's food and cosmetic division said the FDA did not have the information presented by the consumer group when it held the chemicals as "generally recognized as safe."*

When clippings of this release began arriving in the mail from friends and relatives around the country, I was thrilled. The topic that had been of such extreme concern to me was now receiving national exposure. Maybe the FDA would finally act on this issue. God, I hoped so. I was concerned though about their public lie that they had not been alerted to the problems of sulfites in the past. My doctor's first correspondence with the agency dated back to 1977. Well, with Mike Jacobson and the CSPI on my side now, the FDA would have to reconsider the chemical's safety.

One morning in early December, I was listening to Christmas carols on the stereo when my telephone rang and a New York accent addressed me.

"Carolyn Knight, please."

"This is she."

"Hello, Carolyn. This is Esther Kartiganer calling from CBS News. I'm a producer for the '60 Minutes' program and we're exploring the possibility of filming a segment on the uses of sulfiting agents in foods."

I was speechless.

"60 Minutes!" That was the most highly-rated television show in the nation. This was a chance to really get the story told.

I wasn't speechless for long.

21

The "60 Minutes" show wanted to tell the sulfite story! They wanted to expose the chemical's dangers. Millions of people would see such a program and, as dramatic as it might sound, thousands of lives would probably be saved by its airing.

My mind raced. The implications were astronomical. Why, because of the influence and clout of "60 Minutes," the FDA would have no choice but to listen.

"Carolyn, I'd like to fly to California to meet you this weekend," Esther was saying. "I'm also trying to set up appointments with doctors at Scripps Clinic and with another patient who is sulfite sensitive. Would Saturday be convenient for you?"

I laughed to myself. If I'd been expecting the president of the United States for dinner, I would have cancelled his visit for this opportunity.

"Yes, Esther, that would be fine. What time should I expect you?" I couldn't believe how calm and cool I sounded. I gave her directions to Canyon Lake, then hung up and let out a war whoop that would have made Geronimo proud.

I remembered a joke I had heard that says you know it's going to be a bad day when you answer your phone and it's "60 Minutes" calling. But the joke was going to be on the FDA, not on me. I was ecstatic.

My family was equally as excited and teased me all week by referring to me as a movie star.

"Maybe a talent scout will happen to watch and want to give you a screen test," Kathy told me.

"Maybe they'll want to make a movie of your life. Jane Fonda can play you, Mom."

"I want Charles Durning to play me," joked Vick.

"And Brooke Shields can be me," Meri piped in.

"Do you think it would be okay if I offered your producer some of my homemade wine when she's here?" asked Vick.

"What do you want to do, give poor Esther an instant sulfite challenge?" I teased.

We continued bantering throughout the week to overcome our nervous anticipation. But Saturday finally arrived—and with it, Ms. Kartiganer.

A dark-haired, self-assured woman, she interviewed me once again as she had on the phone, looked through the reams of research materials I'd compiled and, yes, had a glass of Vick's wine.

"It looks like this story is one we'd be interested in pursuing," she said before leaving to talk with the other subjects on her list. "I'll present the material to Harry Reasoner on Monday and let you know if it's a go."

From then on I jumped each time the phone rang as I waited for a call from New York. It finally came the following Tuesday.

"Carolyn. Esther here. Harry likes the idea of the story, and we'd like to film you in Canyon Lake next week if that's convenient.

"We'd send a camera crew out on Monday to film a typical day with Carolyn Knight, then Harry would arrive on Wednesday to interview you."

It was really going to happen.

"Of course, Esther. That would be fantastic. But, about this typical day. Mine aren't that exciting. What do you have in mind?"

"I think it would be a good idea to emphasize the fact that you eat only fresh foods," she said. "Do you suppose we could film you shopping for produce at your local market and then at home baking bread or something?"

"Anything you say, Esther. You're the producer. I'll see you Monday."

I hung up and laughed at myself. I was going to be shown on national television going grocery shopping and baking bread. So much for my "career woman" image.

Sleep just wouldn't come Sunday night and, when the alarm rang early Monday morning, I ran to the mirror to inspect myself. I'd just die if I had bags under my eyes as a result of my restless night. Never mind the fact that I'd never had bags in my life. There was a first time for everything.

I stared into the mirror, focusing on the little wrinkles around my eyes and mouth that I preferred to call laugh lines. Nothing I could do about those. My face was a little puffy from the increased cortisone I'd been taking since catching a cold the week before but, all in all, I was content with the face looking back at me.

Stepping into the shower, I welcomed the hot, steamy spray and felt a release of tension as the water coursed over my body. I was as prepared as I'd ever be for the day's excitement. I'd contacted the manager of the grocery store and received permission to bring the camera crew along with me on my shopping spree. I had assured everyone that a mini-cam would probably be used, and that we'd be as unobtrusive as possible as we whisked through the produce department.

I held my head under the shower nozzle and reached for the shampoo, laughing as I remembered my trip to the supermarket the day before. I'd needed a couple of ingredients for the bread I was going to bake in front of the camera, and as I walked through the door, I was surprised to see a group of official-looking men in business suits surveying the produce section.

"Top brass from the L.A. office," the assistant manager whispered to me. "They want to be sure all the apples are polished before you and the '60 Minutes' people arrive tomorrow."

I stepped out of the shower and couldn't help but smile. I wasn't the only one excited about this whole chain of events.

Promptly at 1 p.m. I looked out the window and saw three cars pull up in front of the house. Three cars? How many people did it take to film one person shopping and baking bread?

I soon found out. We caravaned the four miles into the nearest town—with Esther and me leading the way in one car, the camera man and his assistant in another, and the sound man and his equipment in the third. And to think I'd promised the store manager we'd be unobtrusive.

We were anything but.

After asking the manager to turn off the piped-in Christmas music since the segment wouldn't be telecast for a couple of months, the technician wired me for sound. A tiny microphone was attached to my collar and a thin cord was run down the inside of my blouse, out between the last two buttonholes through the belt loops of my skirt and into my pocket, where it was attached to a receiver that had been placed there.

He then strapped a large, heavy-looking machine over his shoulders and, with Esther walking behind him pushing a shopping cart filled with additional sound equipment, the technician was ready to follow me through the store, recording every sigh, cough and wheeze.

Ward and Rick, the cameramen, were busily taking light readings of my face, the apples, the lettuce, the tomatoes and the pineapples, while the other shoppers, their mouths agape, stared at the spectacle we were creating.

I strained my ears to hear some of the comments going on around me.

"They must be filming a commercial."

"No, I understand it's CBS News. I wonder why they're here?"

"The manager told me it's for the '60 Minutes' program."

"Oh, my God. I didn't put on any lipstick."

We were finally ready to roll. I tried to act as natural as possible, but it wasn't easy with the sound man and Esther following behind me, Ward crouched down in front of me, walking backward with the camera whirring and Rick walking backwards behind him holding up a large light.

Acting as nonchalant as possible, I sauntered through the produce aisles, sacking and weighing apples, squeezing heads of lettuce, pinching avocados and picking and choosing the other fruits and vegetables that were so much a part of my diet.

After a few minutes, I began to enjoy my role as television celebrity—as well as the curious glances I was receiving from the other shoppers. I was almost sorry when it was time to make my way through the check-out line and return home to bake bread.

I've never considered myself much of a cook and I felt embarrassed to think my clumsy skills in the kitchen would be telecast into millions of homes.

"You'll probably get letters from housewives all over the country asking where that woman ever learned to bake bread," I told Esther and the crew.

"Hey, it looks great, don't worry," said Ward, and I thought again how kind and considerate he and the rest of the crew were as they sniffed the air and murmured their approval of the warm, yeasty bread dough smell wafting through the house. They were equally as complimentary when they sampled the wheat bread when it came out of the oven and, when we made arrangements to meet again when Harry Reasoner arrived on Wednesday, we said goodbye as friends.

Wednesday dawned a typically bright and sunny December day in Canyon Lake—perfect weather for visiting New Yorkers. Entrances to our private community were secured by guards, and it caused quite a stir when I called the administration office of our homeowners' association and asked them to allow Harry Reasoner and his CBS crew through the gates.

Of all the "60 Minutes" commentators, I had alway liked Harry the best. He had a kind smile and a gentlemanly manner, and I'd been glad to learn it was he who would be interviewing me for the sulfite segment.

I wasn't disappointed. The crew arrived an hour before Harry was expected, to set up the elaborate system of lights, sound equipment and cameras. After walking through the house and rejecting one room after another because of lighting factors and who knows what all, the three men agreed that the best spot for the interview was the kitchen. Another triumph for women's liberation, I thought to myself. But who cared? Reaching millions of homes with the message about sulfur dioxide was the important thing.

Harry and Esther arrived on schedule and were greeted by my whole family. Vick had taken the afternoon off, Kathy was home for the holidays and Meri had just jumped off the school bus. We all hurried outside to greet our famous guest as the car pulled into the driveway.

I held out my hand and welcomed the renowned Mr. Reasoner.

"I can tell already that we're going to get along great," I said, shaking his hand.

The newscaster gave me his quizzical smile and squeezed my hand in return. "And why is that?"

"Because I've always been attracted to older men with silver hair—especially when they're shorter than I am," I quipped, introducing him to my husband.

We all laughed and, with the ice broken, I led everyone into the house.

The interview went smoothly and, thanks to Harry's professionalism and knowledge of the subject, I felt quite at ease throughout the 15-minute question-and-answer period. Actually, I felt as if I could talk the entire day about my experiences with sulfites, but I knew I couldn't monopolize the whole show. Harry still had to talk with my doctor and another patient, as well as with the FDA and my friend at CSPI, Michael Jacobson.

That night, the long-awaited excitement of the day behind us, Vick and I sat in front of the fireplace talking softly. I felt a contentment that I was finding hard to express.

Vick put my feelings into words for me.

"Do you realize what you've done?" he asked. "You've proven that one person really can make a difference in this world of ours. One person *can* fight City Hall."

He cupped my chin in his hands. "I'm so proud of you."

I basked in his praise but knew that I couldn't take all the credit. "You have a hand in this too, you know," I said.

"Me? What did I do?"

"My darling, none of this would have happened if you hadn't tried to woo me with that fatal glass of wine."

22

A roller coaster ride.

That would probably be the best way to describe my life since asthma was first diagnosed in 1972. I'd soar higher and higher with optimism as new theories or discoveries lifted my spirits, then plunge deeply into despair as, one by one, my hopes were dashed.

The euphoria I'd experienced because of the "60 Minutes" program may have taken me higher than I'd ever been, but it wasn't long before I found myself traveling back down that roller coaster track, faster and farther than I'd ever been before.

The ringing of the telephone seemed jarring in the peacefulness of the weekend afternoon. The Sunday paper was strewn over the family room floor, a fire was blazing in our new wood-burning stove and Vick and I were reveling in the opportunity to spend a truly relaxing day together.

Our repose didn't last for long.

I reached for the phone. "Hello?"

"Carolyn, this is Dr. Stevens. I'm sorry to bother you on a Sunday afternoon, but I knew you'd want to be contacted."

I shivered with a sense of foreboding. Despite the fact that Dr. Stevens and I had established a rapport that placed our relationship far beyond that normally found between physician and patient, I was, nonetheless, surprised to hear his voice on the other end of the phone.

"Is something wrong?"

"Carolyn, Jo Valone is in the intensive care unit. She and her husband were eating brunch in a restaurant that advertised 'all fresh foods,' but there must have been sulfites in something she ate."

I was shaking. "How is she now? Is she going to be all right?"

The doctor's voice sounded tired. "She was dead on arrival, but the emergency room staff was able to resuscitate her. She's in a coma and is experiencing grand mal seizures. We're afraid she might have been without oxygen for as long as five to eight minutes."

I fought to hold back the tears. "Is there anything I can do? May I come see her?"

"No one but her husband is allowed to visit her. There's nothing you can do, friend, but I knew you'd want to be informed."

Somehow I managed to thank him for calling and to replace the receiver before completely falling apart.

Loud sobs shook my body and I put my fist to my mouth in an attempt to muffle the sounds I was making. Vick, who had not paid too much attention to the telephone conversation, was at my side in a second, holding me and asking me what was wrong.

I looked at him and shook my head from side to side, unable to speak. I sat in his lap, weeping hysterically until I was completely exhausted and hiccups replaced tears. Then, haltingly, I told him of Dr. Stevens' news.

Vick just hugged me and murmured little sing-song sounds to comfort me. Then, as if the full implication of what had happened finally hit him, he held me at arms length, stared into my red, swollen eyes and swore.

"When is this goddamn government going to do something about this? That could have been you." He once again clutched me to him and we both cried, in sadness for my friend and in fear of the seemingly insurmountable foe—sulfites.

In spite of my doctor's words that there was nothing I could accomplish by being at the hospital, I couldn't stay away. The next morning found me "camped out" in the Intensive Care Unit's waiting room, along with Jo's husband, Bob, and several other relatives. I'd never met Bob before, but we hugged one another as if this tragedy had brought about our instant kinship.

Haggard and exhausted from worry and lack of sleep, Bob sat and retold the frightening story of the circumstances that had occurred the day before.

His shoulders slumped and he twirled his wedding ring around and around his finger as he relived the horror story once again . . . .

Jo and Bob had always enjoyed dining out, though Jo's diet was imited when eating restaurant meals. The couple had found several afes and small eating establishments that were sympathetic to Jo's roblem, and little coffee shop they'd visited that fateful morning had een recommended highly by friends who knew that Jo could eat othing but fresh, unprocessed food.

Despite the claim on the menu that the establishment used fresh roducts, Jo asked her standard question. "Do you use preservatives on our food?"

"No, ma'am. Everything is fresh," said the waitress.

"Now listen, this is very important," Bob interjected, as he always did hen he and Jo ate out. "It's not as if my wife will get a little rash or omething. She could die if she ingests this preservative called sulfite."

The waitress reassured both Bob and Jo. "Everything is brought in esh each day."

Soon the Valones were diving into generous portions of Canadian acon, scrambled eggs and fresh cottage fries.

"It's just great to find another restaurant where we can eat," Jo had just remarked to Bob before her face took on a frightened, stricken look.

"What's wrong, babe?"

Jo stared back at her husband. "I'm not sure, but we'd better go home. I think I'd better use my breathing machine." She sounded short of breath.

Once in the car, Jo's breathing became more labored and she told Bob that they had better head for the hospital instead.

"Hang on, babe. We're on our way. We'll be there in a minute." Bob kept up a constant chatter, trying to assure not only his panicked wife, but himself as well.

Within seconds, however, he stopped talking. Jo had turned blue and her unconscious body was sliding under the dashboard, threatening to interfere with Bob's control of the car.

Speeding down the roadway, ignoring stop signs and traffic signals, Bob voiced a silent prayer and, operating the car with his left hand, attempted to pull Jo's lifeless body back into the passenger side with his right . . . .

"Thank God for the emergency room staff," Bob said to me now, as he paced the small waiting room.

A voice came over the intercom. "Mr. Valone, you may come in now."

Bob turned to me. "Would you like to come back with me?"

"Are you sure they'd allow me to?" I asked.

In answer, Bob took my arm and led me through the double doors of the ward that housed the critically ill patients.

No matter how I'd tried to prepare myself for the eventuality that I might be able to see my friend, nothing could have cushioned my shock.

Jo lay quietly on the hospital bed, her face almost masked completely by the tubes entering her mouth and nose and the electrodes and wires pasted to her head. IVs dripped into both arms, and her hands and feet were flattened to boards to that they would not cramp and twist into claw-like appendages. Huge television-like screens surrounding her monitored her body's every function.

Bob and I stood on either side of the bed, each of us stroking the hand closest to us.

I touched her hair, careful not to disturb any of the wires there. "Oh, Jo," I started in a choked voice, but then realized my tears wouldn't elicit the response I wanted from her.

"Come on, Jo," I started again in a stronger voice. "Hurry up and get out of this bed. We're not going to let them get away with this. We're going to get them this time."

Bob came around and put his arm on my shoulder. Our five minutes were over. We walked together back to the waiting room.

That afternoon I returned home and placed a call to Michael Jacobson in Washington, D.C., to tell him what had happened to Jo. Though he had never met her, his sympathy and concern were sincere, and he was adamant with his advice.

"Carolyn, you're going to have to document the fact that there were sulfites in the food Jo ate. The FDA will not consider this a bona fide case of sulfite poisoning unless it can be proven that the chemical was in something she ate."

"Screw the FDA," I shouted in uncharacteristic abandonment of my normally professional, business-like manner. "You and I both know there must have been sulfites in those potatoes. The only documentation the FDA is going to believe is dead people."

"Now, Carolyn, I know this situation with your friend is very upsetting, but we've got to be practical. Do you know of anyone who could go back to that restaurant and order those potatoes so that we can chemically analyze them?"

The hair on the back of my neck bristled as I considered the chore that lay before me. "Yes, I know of someone who will do it—I will."

I could almost feel Mike's hand patting me on the back to give me strength, despite the fact that he was 3000 miles away.

The next morning as I showered, I tried to think up excuses I could give the waitress so that I could get those potatoes out of the restaurant. I was afraid the little establishment was already on guard—after all, it was no secret that Jo was ill when she'd left there, and Dr. Stevens had called the manager to ask what preservatives were used in food that had placed one of his patients at death's door.

But it was absolutely imperative that I get a sample of those potatoes. I continued to play various scenarios in my mind as I got dressed and drove the 60 miles to the now infamous coffee shop. It was nearing 11 a.m. when I got there. In my nervousness I had made several wrong turns. Would they still be serving breakfast? Oh, God, please let me pull this off.

I parked my car in front of the building and couldn't help but notice the hand-made signs taped to every available inch of window space, touting the restaurant's fresh food menu and low prices. I sighed with relief to see one that said, "We serve breakfast all day."

I bought a newspaper to give me something to do while I waited for my breakfast, then took a deep breath, walked into the restaurant and chose a single table in the back of the dining room.

"I was glad to see your sign advertising breakfast all day long," I told the waitress as she approached. "I left Riverside early this morning and didn't take time to eat, and now I feel shaky, so I'm glad you serve breakfast."

Oh, God, don't overdo it, I told myself. Stop rattling on. Try to act natural.

I ordered the same breakfast Jo had ordered two days before, then asked the waitress—casually I hoped—if there were preservatives in the potatoes.

"No, everything is fresh."

The waitress left and I opened the paper—not to read, but to hide behind. I couldn't believe they were sticking to their "freshness" story despite Jo's reaction and the doctor's inquiries.

Within minutes an over-sized plate of eggs, bacon and potatoes was placed before me and I gave the waitress a half-hearted smile as I contemplated what to do next. I didn't dare put any of it in my mouth, yet I had told the waitress I was shaky from the lack of food.

I pushed the mass of eggs back and forth on my plate, trying to decide what to do. The potatoes took up at least a third of my plate and, I had to admit, did look fresh. Instead of the perfectly uniform slices one would expect of frozen or processed fries, these resembled the fried potatoes I'd make at home—alternately thick and thin pieces that looked as if they'd just been sliced in the kitchen, as the waitress had implied.

Noticing that I hadn't taken a bite, the young woman walked to my table and asked if the food was cooked to my liking.

"Oh, yes. It's fine. But, I just remembered an appointment I must keep. Could I have this to go?" I asked, handing her my plate.

She returned several minutes later with my breakfast in a styrofoam container and, once I had "the evidence" in my hands, I asked to see the manager.

"Is something wrong?"

"I'm not sure," I replied. "I want to ask him about the potatoes."

"The manager won't be in until this afternoon, but would you like to see the cook?"

I said I would and, when I reached the kitchen, my eyes were drawn immediately to a large, clear plastic bag full of cut white potatoes sitting on the counter.

"Are those potatoes preserved in any way?" I asked.

Busy flipping pancakes on the grill, the cook nonchalantly glanced at me. "I don't know. You'd have to ask the distributor."

My cheeks began to burn in anger, and I struggled to hold my tongue. How could anyone be so stupid as to think those potatoes were fresh as the waitress had assured me—and Jo. Anyone knows that sliced potatoes don't stay white for very long. Unless they're preserved, they turn a brownish-gray color.

I wrote down the name and phone number of the distributor, jumped in my car and tried not to break the speed limit as I drove to my mother's and dad's house several miles away. I wanted to get those potatoes in a freezer fast, as Mike Jacobson had instructed me to.

Later, the "poisoned potatoes" safely tucked away in my parents' freezer, I called the number given me for the distributor.

"I don't know anything about preservatives," he said. "I'm just the jobber who buys products from Farm Fresh and sells them to a bunch of little mom and pop places in the area."

Passing the buck, he gave me the number of his distributor, who answered the line on the first ring.

"I'm interested in finding out if there are any preservatives in the cottage fresh fries you sell," I told them.

"Well, of course there are," he said, with almost a sneer in his voice as if I'd asked the most stupid question in the world.

"What preservative do you use?"

"It's called bi-sulfite."

Despite the fact that I had known all along that would be his answer, I felt shocked and unable to believe that people so matter-of-factly used a chemical that had the potential of being so deadly.

I replaced the receiver quietly, then turned to my mom and dad.

"Mission accomplished," I said.

Jo remained in a coma for more than a month before her eyes fluttered open and she began to respond to the people around her. The neurologist thought it was a miracle, but I knew better. It was love—and I told Bob so.

"I've never seen a more devoted husband," I said to him one night on the phone when he called to give me a progress report. "You never left the hospital even though they only let you see her five minutes of every hour. I know it was your love that kept Jo alive."

Bob's voice was quiet and almost shy as he answered modestly, "Well, that's my baby in there, you know."

After two months in the hospital, Jo was moved to a rehabilitation center to undergo extensive therapy for the brain damage she had suffered—all because she had believed the word "fresh" on a restaurant menu.

So far my crusade hadn't been as successful as I'd hoped. I hadn't been able to save my friend. Who would be next?

23

You have performed an outstanding public service by revealing your experience with sulfiting agents . . . ."

"By extreme coincidence, the day before your program, my wife collapsed in a restaurant . . . ."

"Both my husband and brother-in-law have severe allergies, and my brother-in-law has gone into anaphylactic shock after eating vegetable soup . . . ."

"My uncle died at 42 after eating a meal in a restaurant. The doctors diagnosed it as cardiac arrest, but his death has always been held in suspicion . . . ."

"I always wheeze after drinking white wine. Do you think I might be allergic to sulfites?"

For weeks after the "60 Minutes" show aired, I was flooded with mail and calls from people all over the United States who had related my experience to their own. They came from people who were strictly interested in nutrition as well as from those who were undoubtedly afflicted by sufiting agents.

After the program, the National Restaurant Association advised its members to refrain from using sulfites or to inform their patrons if the chemical was being used by their establishments. I felt that strides were finally being made—and knew that the issue was really gaining momentum when Paul Harvey featured a segment on the chemical's dangers on his nationally syndicated radio program.

Newspapers, radio stations and other television programs were interested also, and I had the opportunity to tell my story again and again. I encouraged others who thought they might be sulfite sensitive to contact the FDA and, within a short time, 90 additional complaints had been registered with the consumer safety officer there.

Surprisingly, thirty percent of the complaints were from non-asthmatics, from people who had suffered from gastro-intestinal symptoms, headaches, hives, and other illnesses after ingesting sulfite-saturated foods. In addition, restaurant workers who came into contact with the chemical complained of rashes on their hands and arms from encountering sulfiting solutions.

But consumers weren't the only ones inundating the federal agency with mail—the food industry was making its voice heard too, and it was a voice that expressed outrage and concern that their profits would be affected and the shelf life of their products shortened if this widely used preservative were banned.

> *Sulfur dioxide fumigation is essential to the marketing, transport, storage and export of table grapes,* wrote the California Grape and Treefruit League. *There is no known substitute for the gaseous compound that is effective in preventing mold-rot and other storage fungi and that prolongs storage life.*
>
> *Restriction or removal of the use of SO_2 on fresh grapes will impact the entire industry, valued at $400 million. Consumers, as well as growers-packers-shippers, will suffer from reduced availability and quality.*
>
> *On behalf of California's fresh grape industry, it is the League's recommendation that sulfiting agents be affirmed by the FDA as generally recognized as safe.*

Not surprisingly, the wine industry sent an eleven-page document disputing the claims that sulfur dioxide was dangerous.

> *The results of a study by Dr. Vincent Marinkovich proved convincingly that there were no life-threatening reactions to asthmatics who were sensitive to sulfur dioxide,* said the report. *The opponents to the use of sulfur dioxide cleverly confuse their data. They speak of 'reactions occurring after the ingestion of certain restaurant foods and wine.' The point which they miss is the fact that the restaurant foods discussed were certain salads which had been sprayed with sulfite salts to prevent the fruits or vegetables from browning, and that the atmosphere above these certain fruits and vegetables contain sulfur dioxide per se. It is not the sulfur dioxide which had been disolved in the wine which resulted in the conditions claimed but rather the sulfur dioxide gas in the atmosphere of the sprayed vegetables. When taken orally, disolved in a product such as wine, sulfur dioxide is harmless.*
>
> *. . . An assumption was made that the sulfite on the salad might have been responsible for the anaphylaxis and tests were performed after the fact. Certainly the lives and activities of 200 million people should not be regulated because one person allegedly required emergency medical aid due to assumed sulfur dioxide on his salad . . . .*

> *The Biscuit and Cracker Manufacturers' Association is the national trade association of the cookie and cracker industry. Its members manufacture approximately 85*

percent of the total production of cookies and crackers in the United States. This industry has been for many years, and continues to be, a substantial user of sodium sulfite in the manufacture of its products.

Sodium sulfite is widely used by our industry to provide machinability of doughs by causing the protein to relax, thereby moving the dough more readily through the equipment.

Its safety in food use may be accepted without question on the basis of centuries of use. It is accordingly requested that the FDA recognize the need for and the use of sodium sulfite by the cookie and cracker industry and not remove it from GRAS status.

Mrs. Smith's Frozen Foods Co., a wholly owned subsidiary of the Kellogg Company, is a leading producer of frozen and fresh baked pies and pie dough in addition to other frozen products which include crepes, quiche, Italian entrees, waffles and waffle batter.

It is believed that the proposed specific limitations with respect to use of sodium bisulfite and sodium metabisulfite as direct human food ingredients are unjustified by available scientific evidence, would unduly restrain improvements in the food supply by inhibiting innovations and improvements in manufacturing, and represent an improper attempt to regulate these substances as food additives under the guise of the GRAS affirmation provisions.

Sodium bisulfite is a critical and necessary ingredient in our frozen pie shells, frozen pies, frozen cobblers and other dough products, wrote Contech Laboratories Pet Incorporated. *These are major product lines for our company which are enjoyed by a great number of consumers. We know of no allowable substitute which will provide the desired functional effect of sodium bisulfite in this type of product. Restricting the usage level would jeopardize some of our major profitable product lines as well as the jobs of a considerable number of our employees.*

Our company is and has been using sodium metabisulfite as an agent in processing instant tea products, wrote Tetley, Inc. *The consumer has come to expect an instant tea beverage which is bright reddish in color and clear in appearance. However, the beverage produced from an extract, untreated with a processing agent, is dull in color and muddy in appearance. In order to obtain consumer acceptance of the instant tea beverage, we use sodium metabisulfite as a processing agent.*

The ocean quahog clam represents an important new food (protein) source which can be made commercially and popularly acceptable by the use of a sodium bisulfite treating agent, wrote the National Fisheries Institute. *The proposed regulation of sulfiting agents would prohibit sodium bisulfite from being used as described and may eliminate the ocean quahog clam as a food source.*

Was the future of the clam more important than the future of sulfite-sensitive members of the population? I guess I'd been naive enough to believe that, when the chemical's danger was brought to its attention, the food industry would find substitutes for sulfur dioxide.

Many companies were even fighting a proposal to label products. It would cost too much, they complained. Now, I had been dealing with printers for years, and I knew that changing the wording on a label would incur minimal costs. The industry didn't worry about changes in labeling if they were adding words such as "new" or "improved."

Many of the industry letters to the FDA stated that sulfites in processed foods dissipated by the time the product reached the consumer's table. However, my own reactions belied that contention. My lungs knew better! And my belief was supported by a study of the amounts of sulfur dioxide that could be recovered from food using a procedure called the Monier-William distillation method. During an evaluation of the procedure by the FDA's Division of Chemistry and Physics, foods were spiked with varying amounts of sulfites and then tested to see how much of the chemical could be recovered. In some foods, such as grapes, dried fruits and lemon juice, the recovery level was about 90 percent. However, in other foods such as broccoli, avocado dip, crackers and potato chips, only a small percentage of the sulfiting agent could be recovered.

What happened to the rest? "The reduced recoveries are due to reactive components in the food matrix which irreversibly react with sulfites," said the FDA report.

But the chemical was *still* in the food, despite the technician's inability to account for it. I was living proof of that—and had almost been dead proof several times.

The controversy continued to grow, and most of the time it seemed that "the other side" seemed to tip the scales.

"The public shouldn't stew over food additives," read the headline of one newspaper account, reporting the quotes of a so-called health expert who preached that Americans made too much fuss about sugar, salt and food additives.

Dr. Edwin M. Foster told members of the American Dietetic Association that the American public is at "near hysteria" about additives which, he said, never hurt anyone. A professor of food microbiology at the University of Wisconsin and the director of the Food Research Institute, Foster said the "gullible public should stop worrying about the hypothetical and imaginary dangers.

"I can never recall a documented incident of illness from any approved food additive," he said to 10,000 convention goers—and his uneducated views were appearing on the first page of major newspapers around the country!

Equally upsetting was a syndicated column by a so-called wine expert that appeared nationwide.

> **Q.** *I was hospitalized recently for what apparently was an allergic reaction to chemical additives in wine. Since then I have heard of cases in which allergic reactions similar to mine have resulted in death. I also heard that, in tests conducted at a leading medical center, the sulfur dioxide used in winemaking was found responsible. Do you have any information on the subject?*
>
> **A.** *Several things about your letter puzzle me. Indeed, were I of suspicious bent, I might conjecture that you are ideologically opposed to wine (and other beverages that contain alcohol) and have fabricated your case history for political purposes.*
>
> *In any event, conjectures about motives aside, I cannot comment intelligently on second- or third-hand reports of alleged deaths resulting from alleged allergic reactions among people who allegedly drank wine . . . .*

I was appalled at this wine expert's attitude. Some poor person had written him for information that might help save his or her life and was answered in a rude, belligerent and misinformed manner.

I was angry all over again. It seemed that the sulfite situation took one step forward and three steps backward.

I remembered recent newspaper articles, and even a movie made for TV, about a woman who had formed a group called MADD, Mothers Against Drunk Drivers. She had made headway by organizing. Perhaps that's what all of us who were sulfite-sensitive should do.

Again, as if my thoughts worked magic, I received a call from a woman whose son had reacted violently to sulfited food in a restaurant. She had almost lost the young man in the emergency room after the incident and, like a mother lion whose cub is threatened, Dale Norman was ready to go for the jugular.

"I think we should form a consumers' advocacy group," she said. "Would you be willing to help?"

Would I!

It was just the encouragement I needed. I finally had an ally—one that was as deeply concerned and as eager to get involved as I.

"Let's call ourselves SO_2S for Stamp Out Sulfites," I suggested the next time we talked. "No one will have to know there are only two of us."

I suddenly had the feeling that with our determination and tenacity, the team of Knight and Norman could do the work of 200.

24

I glanced at my mother and squeezed her hand. Together we began climbing the long stone ladder of steps leading to the imposing federal building in Los Angeles.

Dale Norman and I, as representatives of Stamp Out Sulfites, had been placed on the agenda for the FDA's consumer exchange meeting. None of the other sulfite-sensitive persons could take the time to attend the meeting with us, so my mother and Dale's mother and husband had agreed to accompany us. Not only would they provide moral support, but they would also sign in as SO_2S supporters, which we hoped would give our fledgling organization more credibility.

"Mom, this is crazy, but I'm more nervous about this than I was about the '60 Minutes' show. I'm not very good at public speaking."

"Now, you'll do just fine, as you always do." She took my hand again. "Don't worry."

That was my mother. Always positive that I'd succeed at anything I tried. I was glad she had come.

As we walked into the lobby I spotted Dale, looking calm and in control.

"We're first on the agenda," she told me as we greeted one another and introduced our family members. She pointed to the grocery sack I carried. "What's in the bag?"

"Oh, just some packaged food I brought along to help me make a point."

We entered the conference room and took seats in the front row. I reached toward the head table and took one of the handouts placed there. It was an FDA "Talk Paper," a bulletin prepared by the Office of Public Affairs "to guide FDA personnel in responding with consistency and accuracy to questions from the public on subjects of current interest."

By coincidence this particular issue was entitled "Sulfiting Agents" and referred to the "60 Minutes" program, centering on the fact that the FDA was reviewing the chemical's GRAS status. The last sentence jarred me.

"Dale, listen to this. 'The agency reminds allergy-prone consumers that these sulfiting agents, when used, are listed on the ingredients labeling of packaged foods.' If they believe that, we've got a bigger problem on our hands than we thought."

Before she could reply the meeting was called to order—and all of a sudden, I felt ready. My initial fear had been replaced by indignation, and I couldn't wait to take the floor.

Within minutes Dale and I were facing the audience and our first public forum as consumer advocates.

"The FDA was created more than 75 years ago to protect consumers from products that could endanger their health," I began. "However, there are currently as many as one million asthmatics who are threatened each day by products that are recognized as safe by the FDA. Those products are called sulfiting agents, and we're here today to ask you to take action on these highly dangerous chemicals."

Dale and I then proceeded to discuss the uses of sulfites in restaurant foods, processed foods and medicines used primarily for asthmatics.

"A major problem concerning sulfiting agents is that many of the medications used to control asthma are preserved with this chemical," Dale told the gathering. "Asthmatics who have ingested sulfiting agents in a restaurant situation and who are rushed to an emergency center will most assuredly be injected with drugs containing this preservative."

Her voice became stronger as she listed the many drugs given to asthma-sufferers that could in reality finish the deadly job a restaurant meal began.

"The FDA must ban the use of SO_2 in medicines for asthmatics at once, and emergency personnel throughout the United States should be alerted immediately to the potentially life-threatening situation of sulfite sensitive asthmatics who may enter their institutions in need of emergency care."

I studied the audience as Dale spoke. I knew that the only ones here who had heard of sulfites before were probably the people we had brought with us. Yet the entire group was sitting on the edge of their seats. It was *their* food that was being adulterated, also. The restaurant foods they ate were spiked with chemicals, too.

I reached into my "bag of tricks" as I approached the podium and held up the Talk Paper I had grabbed when we first sat down.

"The FDA is either lying or is sorely misinformed," I began. The audience gasped, and even my mother looked surprised at my harsh words.

"In the agency's recent bulletin it is recommended that asthmatics read the labels of foods they buy since sulfites are listed as ingredients if they are used. I want to dispute that claim."

I held up a bottle of catsup and read its ingredients to those assembled. The first ingredient listed was "red, ripe tomatoes," I told them.

"In his definitive study, 'Sulfur Dioxide: Its Application in Foods, Beverages and Pharmaceuticals,' Dr. Louis Schroeter discusses a patented procedure used to keep ripe tomatoes in a fresh condition for indefinite periods of time," I said, my voice strong and unwavering.

"That procedure involves soaking tomatoes in a sulfite solution for as long as *four years*. Yet the use of sulfites is never listed on any tomato product."

I held up the catsup bottle again. "How are we to know whether the 'red, ripe tomatoes' that are listed on this label are red, ripe tomatoes that have been soaked for years in a substance that is poison to many asthmatics?"

I had them now. People were turning to one another, murmuring at this insight into food processing methods.

I bent down and snatched a box of cornstarch from the bag I had brought.

"This box of cornstarch lists no ingredients at all," I said. "But it does use the words 'pure' and 'wholesome' and says 'It is carefully manufactured by modern processes from fully ripened corn.' "

I glanced from one side of the room to the other. "Would you like to hear about those modern processes? Dr. Theron Randolph has researched the use of chemicals in our food supply and says that the processing of corn begins with the soaking of the whole kernel in a sulfur dioxide solution. That prevents fermentation of the corn while it is being processed. But it also imparts sulfur contamination to all manufactured corn products—corn meal, corn flour, corn syrup, corn oil and, yes, this cornstarch."

The FDA officials were fidgeting and looking uncomfortable, but I ignored them and continued my tirade.

"Corn and tomatoes are just two small examples that illustrate the uses of SO_2," I said. "The chemical is the most widely used preservative in our nation, yet most of you have probably never heard of it until today. Why? Ask them," I said, pointing to the FDA officials.

"And if corrupting our food supply isn't bad enough, consider this—most food packaging paper is sulfited, also, to help the products retain their 'freshness.' And while the FDA *has* prohibited the use of sulfites in meats, butcher paper itself is highly sulfited to keep meats from turning brown or gray.

"That, ladies and gentlemen, is deception. It's unjust and, in my opinion, immoral. And, in the cases of people such as myself and Dale Norman's son, it could also be lethal."

I then proceeded to tell the story of Jo Valone before I sat down and released the podium to Dale once again. In her no-nonsense manner she listed demands of SO_2S.

"We want an immediate ban on the use of sulfiting agents in restaurants as well as their use as preservatives in medicines used for asthmatics," she said. "And we recommend the FDA require immediate labeling of all products containing sulfites, including the application of the chemical early in the distribution process, such as by packers, processors and wholesalers.

"SO_2S is deeply concerned about this issue and thanks you for giving us the opportunity to bring this important matter to your attention," she said in closing. "The matter is in your hands now, and nothing must delay those immediate actions which are necessary to save unknown sulfite sufferers from serious respiratory distress or even death."

Dale picked up her notes and I rose to meet her as she walked toward me. We gave our SO_2S supporters the high sign and they rose also to walk toward the door.

"Thank you, ladies. You've made a very strong statement," said the chairman in a placatory, yet non-committal voice as we wended our way through the rows of folded chairs.

As we left, the occupants of those chairs smiled, grasped our hands, told us good luck and even asked us for business cards. We'd made quite an impact here—but would that impact be felt in Washington where it could do some good?

Not soon enough, I discovered the next day, when I received a call from Michael Jacobson, from the Center for Science in the Public Interest.

"Carolyn, are you sitting down? I have some bad news. The first death that can be directly linked to sulfites has just occurred."

25

A man had died.

A fellow asthma sufferer had died because of SO_2.

He'd been eating a meal with his family in a Mexican restaurant somewhere in Arizona and had died of anaphylactic shock right before their eyes.

A husband had died.

A father had died.

He'd been rushed to the emergency ward and had been injected with drugs preserved with the very chemical that had sent him there in the first place.

I put my head on my desk and cried, sobbing as if I'd lost my own father, for I did feel a kinship to this unknown man. I knew what his last few minutes of life had been like. I shared his agony.

How many others had there been? How many more would there have to be before the FDA gave the subject more than lip service?

I walked into the bathroom, blew my nose and turned on the faucet, cupping the cold water in my hands and splashing my face. Avoiding the reflection of my red eyes and blotchy cheeks, I quickly dried my face and returned to my office.

I opened my file and grasped the bulging file of letters from others who had written of their sulfite-induced experiences. I needed to read them again. I felt so close to all of them, though most of us had never met. We all lived such precarious lives. What had happened to our friend in Arizona could have happened to any of us.

I sifted through my letters and reread the one from a young man in Maryland.

> *I almost died from eating a salad at a restaurant in Gaithersburg, Maryland. I had prepared a salad at the salad bar. About five minutes after finishing the salad, I started having difficulty breathing. I am an asthmatic, so I was able to administer Bronkosol through a nebulizer I always carried with me. It had no effect at all.*
>
> *I quickly realized I was having a very bad attack. I was fighting for air. I asked the manager of the restaurant to*

call an ambulance. Within three minutes I was unconscious and had stopped breathing completely.

Fortunately, the paramedics were stationed just a few blocks away. In the ambulance, I was given an injection of epinephrine, which my doctor said probably saved my life. I was rushed to the hospital where I regained consciousness in the emergency room.

The doctors had no idea what had caused the attack. They told me I was lucky to be alive and that it was fortunate I had suffered no brain damage, since I had stopped breathing for a significant length of time. I remained in intensive care for three days and in a regular room in the hospital for another two days.

After I was discharged, my allergist determined I was very likely sensitive to sulfiting agents. However, because my doctor feared I might have an even more serious reaction, he decided not to risk testing the degree of my sensitivity.

Since my attack, I've learned that sulfiting agents are used in salads, seafood and frozen foods. It's even used in my asthma medication, Bronkosol.

I've also learned that the Food and Drug Administration thinks sulfiting agents are safe. FDA thinks all that is necessary is a sign in restaurants saying 'sodium bisulfite added.' Any sign like that wouldn't have helped me, because I didn't know before the attack that I was senstive to sulfiting agents.

A fellow asthma sufferer who I had met at Scripps Clinic wrote of a recent experience he'd had:

. . . I probably shouldn't have walked to the restaurant that night. There was an inversion layer holding the automobile exhaust on the ground like a lid holds steam in a pot. I was already short of breath when I was seated at the restaurant and the fish entree I ordered, unbeknowst to me, had been treated with sulfites.

As you know, Carolyn, I carry adrenalin with me just as you do. I knew I was in trouble so I made my way to the men's room, but my hands were shaking so much that I dropped the vial. It broke on the tile floor before I could fill my syringe. God, I was panicked.

Two other men came into the restroom just then and I tried to ask them to get help. They saw the syringe in my hand and assumed I was a dope addict—can you believe that? They just told me to stay away from them.

I was losing consciousness, I could tell. Another man came in and all I could do was hold out my hand to him and gasp, "Please . . . doctor." He left, too, but evidently found a phone and called an ambulance. The next thing I knew I was in the hospital emergency room.

Another letter caught my eye, from a young woman who had written of an equally harrowing experience:

> *I'd gone out with this nice guy and accepted his invitation for a nightcap in his apartment. That 'nightcap' was a bottle of wine and, as I drank a glass of it, I could feel my lungs begin to tighten. I told my date I wasn't feeling well and left as fast as I could. I got all the way to my car before I realized I was in big trouble.*
>
> *I decided I'd better go back and ask my new friend to get help. He lived in an upstairs apartment, and I don't know how I ever climbed those stairs! I managed to get to his door, but passed out before I could ring his doorbell. Luckily, he was still in the living room and heard a thump (me falling), opened the door and called the paramedics.*
>
> *Needless to say, that was my last date with him.*

I smiled at her sense of humor. But the situation was not funny. It had taken on new proportions. One of us had died.

My despair continued over the next few days as I tried to think of some new way to approach the problem of sulfiting agents. I'd fought them for more than 12 years, first as an unknown enemy, then as foe that seemed to grow larger than Goliath as the years passed. Now I felt even smaller than David—and the stones I'd cast were merely pebbles, falling much too short of their target.

Hearing from the daughter of the Arizona man who had died only deepened my depression.

> *We knew he had a reaction to something he ate, but we didn't know what it was. It shouldn't have happened. My father didn't have to die that day in front of us. The food he ate at that restaurant was treated with sulfiting agents.*
>
> *My mother, brother and I were robbed of my dad. If dad had known about sulfiting agents he would still be here today.*
>
> *Please help me tell the FDA to ban sulfiting agents. I don't want to see this happen to anyone else . . .*

I didn't want to see it happen to anyone else, either. But what more could I do? When I discovered my allergy to sulfites I'd opened a Pandora's box.

It seemend that every time I thought I'd made some headway down the path to a solution, a dozen roadblocks appeared in my way.

Maybe I wasn't cut out for this consumer advocacy role in which I'd found myself.

I wasn't a crusader.

I wasn't a politician.

I wasn't a lobbyist.

I was just a writer.

As if that proverbial light bulb turned on over my head, I knew what I had to do. Yes, I was a writer and, as all writers know, the pen is mightier than the sword.

I hurried into my office, rolled a sheet of paper into the typewriter and began to type:

Gasping for breath, I made my way into the ladies room and sought refuge in one of the cramped metal cubicles . . . .

Epilogue

At the time *Canary In A Coal Mine* was published, seven deaths had been documented as having been sulfite related, and dozens of other cases were being investigated. The Food and Drug Administration, founded to protect consumers from products that could be hazardous to their health, had still not acted. How many must die before the FDA accepts its responsibility?

What Are Sulfiting Agents

Sulfiting Agents (sulfur dioxide, potassium bisulfite, potassium metabisulfite, sodium bisulfite, sodium metabisulfite, and sodium sulfite) have been used for centuries as sanitizing agents for food containers and fermentation equipment, as preservatives and as anti-oxidants to inhibit browning and discoloration in foods during preparation, storage and distribution. The Food and Drug Administration considers them "generally recognized as safe," and as such, the chemicals are exempted from premarketing clearances required for food additives. The use of sulfiting agents has increased dramatically in the past 10 years—especially in processed and restaurant foods.

Do You Think You Might Be Allergic To Sulfites?

After eating "fresh" fruits and vegetables, salads, potatoes in restaurants—after drinking beer or wine—or after eating dried fruits—have you ever felt flush, faint, weak? Experienced severe wheezing, chest tightness, shortness of breath or loss of consciousness? These symptoms are classic for those asthmatics allergic to sulfiting agents. Doctors estimate that perhaps as many as one in 10 asthmatics is affected in this way and that deaths and comas have occurred. However, asthmatics aren't the only ones affected, and 30% of the people filing complaints with the FDA have exhibited other manifestations of sulfite syndrome, including hives, gastro-intestinal problems and headaches.

If you believe you may be reacting to these dangerous substances, contact your doctor or one of the few centers in the United States now conducting "sulfite challenges."

Dr. Ronald Simon
Scripps Clinic
10666 North Torrey Pines Rd.
La Jolla, CA 92037
619/455-9100

Dr. John Selner
National Jewish Hospital
Denver, CO
303/232-6475

Dr. Metcalf
National Institute of Health
Washington, D.C.
Contact: Marilyn Hinnenkamp
301/496-2785

Dr. Robert Bush
University of Wisconsin Hospital
Madison, WI
608/263-6180

Avoiding Sulfites

The FDA lists the following categories of foods in which sulfiting agents may be used:

Baked Goods and Baking Mixes including all ready-to-eat and ready-to-bake products, flours, and mixes requiring preparation before serving.

Cookies, crackers, crepes, mixes with dried fruits or dried vegetables, pie crusts, pizza crusts, quiche crusts, soft pretzels, tortillas, tortilla shells and waffles.

Alcoholic Beverages including beer, wine, cocktail mixes.

Non-Alcoholic Beverages and Beverage Bases including cola and fruit types, instant tea, tea bags, fruit and vegetable flavored gelatin drinks.

Condiments and Relishes including horseradish relish, onion relish, pickle relish, pickles, olives, salad dressing mixes, wine vinegars.

Confections and Frostings including brown sugar, raw sugar, powdered sugar, marshmallows.

Fish Products processed, frozen, canned and dried clams, shrimp, lobster, crab, scallops, dried cod.

Fresh Fish including clams, shrimp, lobster, crab and scallops.

Fresh Fruit including fruit salad bars, fruit in salads and delis, grapes (which are stored after being sprayed with SO_2 to keep them fresh even out of season).

Fresh Vegetables including salad bars, mushrooms, avocado salad and guacamole, shredded cabbage such as cole slaw, potato products.

Gelatins, Puddings, and Fillings including fruit fillings, flavored gelatins, pectin jelling agents and unflavored gelatin.

Grain Products and Pastas including corn starch, modified food starch, spinach, pasta, breadings, batters, noodle and rice mixes.

Gravies and Sauces including packaged and canned (milk-based included).

Hard Candies

Jams and Jellies

Nuts and Nut Products including shredded coconut.

Plant Protein Products such as soy protein.

Processed Fruits and Fruit Juices including canned, bottled or frozen fruit juices (including lemon, lime, grape, apple and orange). Dried fruit, including apples, apricot, pineapple, peaches, pears, golden raisins, prunes. Canned, bottled or frozen dietetic fruit and fruit juices. Maraschino cherries and glazed fruits.

Processed Vegetables and Vegetable Juices including juices, canned vegetables, pickled vegetables, such as sauerkraut, cauliflower and peppers, dried vegetables, instant mashed potatoes, frozen vegetables and deli potato salads and vegetable salads.

Snack Foods including dried fruit snacks, trail mixes, filled crackers, tortilla chips, corn chips, potato chips.

Soups and Soup Mixes including canned seafood soups and dried soup mixes.

White Granulated Sugar

Sweet Sauces, Toppings and Syrups including corn syrups, maple syrups, fruit toppings, high fructose corn syrup and pancake syrup.

Note: Though sulfiting agents are probably the most widely-used preservatives in processed foods, their use almost never appears on labels, so beware!

Beware of **Catered Foods, Buffets, Cafeteria Establishments.** Ask your produce manager if the fresh produce is sprayed with a sulfite solution. In restaurants, avoid fresh fruits, vegetables, avocado dishes, potatoes—even if the restaurant itself has not added a sulfiting agent, it is most probable that it was added during the storage or shipment process.

Pharmaceuticals

Perhaps the most distressing use of sulfiting agents is as preservatives in drugs used for asthmatics. The following prescription medications designed for respiratory sufferers include dangerous sulfur dioxide preservatives: Bronkosol, Isoprel, Alupent, Decadron, Adrenalin cloride, Metoclopramide hydrochloride, Micronefrin, Dopamine, Celestone suluspan, Hydrocortone Phosphate, Hydrocortone Acetate, Decadron Phosphate, Hexadrol Phosphate, Hydeltrasol and Decadron Phosphate with Xylocaine. In addition, many I.V. solutions, injectable and liquified medications are preserved with sulfites to keep them from discoloring. Buy a PHYSICIAN'S DESK REFERENCE, which lists ingredients of all drugs, and check every medication before you take it.

Environmental Uses

Asthmatics who are sulfite-sensitive must also be aware of environmental uses for SO_2. It is a by-product of coal burning, electric generating power plants, oil refineries, wood pulp production plants. It is a major component of smog, acid rain and acid fog. SO_2 is used in manufacturing rubber, steel, paints, explosives, rayon and detergents. It is used in many spa and pool cleaners and is emitted from kerosene heaters so popular in many of today's homes. Sulfite-sensitive persons have also been known to have attacks from licking envelopes chemically treated with sulfiting agents.

Help Yourself

Wear a Medic Alert bracelet stating your allergy to sulfiting agents and warning emergency personnel not to give drugs preserved with the chemicals. Bracelets and emblems may be ordered from "Medic Alert Foundation," Post Office Box 1009, Turlock, California 95381.

Carry an information sheet in your wallet, in your car—and ask your family members to do the same in case they may be with you when your require emergency care—stating your sensitivity and drugs you *may* and *may not* have.

Ask your doctor to prescribe a kit that includes an adrenalin injection so you may treat yourself when life-threatening attacks occur away from medical help.

There is some indication that Vitamin B_{12} helps to block the extreme reactions asthmatics have to sulfiting agents. However, just as each individual's tolerance to sulfites differs, so does the dose needed to block the attacks. Talk to your doctor about the safety of the B vitamin in your case.

Visit your local hospital emergency room during the time when the staff can sit down with you and listen to your concerns. Explain to them that if you are brought in during an attack that there are medications normally given in emergency respiratory situations that could probably take your life. A caring hospital will enter this information in their medical records computer files, giving you an extra margin of safety if aid is required at their particular facility.

Help SO_2S Fight These Dangerous Chemicals!

STAMP OUT SULFITES (SO_2S) was founded in 1983 by Carolyn Knight and Dale Norman to pressure local and federal agencies and the food and restaurant industries to stop the indiscriminate uses of sulfiting agents. Most uses of sulfites are for cosmetic reasons and deceive the public into believing they are receiving *fresh* foods. Actually, lettuce in restaurants can be kept crisp and green indefinitely by spraying or soaking in sulfiting preservatives. THIS IS FRAUD! This is adulteration of the food supply. And, there is more and more evidence that it is also life-threatening to hundreds of thousands of people.

Stamp Out Sulfites (SO_2S) has made the following demands to the FDA:

- Ban the use of sulfites in restaurant foods.
- If sulfites were used at any time in the distribution process of restaurant foods, such uses must be mentioned on the restaurant menu.
- Ban the use of sulfites in drugs designed for asthmatics and review the uses of the preservatives in all other prescribed medications.
- Review the widespread use of sulfites in processed foods and *label* all products in which sulfites are used in any form or at any time during the processing, storage or distribution.

Please add your voice by contacting the following agencies and legislators:

Dr. Mary Custer
FDA, Bureau of Foods
Divison of Food and Color Additives (HFF-335)
200 C. Street, S.W.
Washington, D.C. 20204
202/426-9463

(Mary Custer is presently writing a proposal on the stand the FDA should take on the sulfiting issue.)

Senator Albert Gore
Washington D.C.

Congressman Ted Weiss
Washington, D.C.

FDA
Epidemiological Investigations (HF-510)
5600 Fishers Lane
Rockville, Maryland 20857
301/443-4667
(This department is currently collecting data on adverse reactions to sulfites)

Rep. Henry Waxman
Chairman, House Sub-committee on Health and the Environment
Washington, D.C.
(Emphasize the FDA's failure to act. Send letter to attention of Bill Corr.)

National Restaurant Association
311 First Street, N.W.
Washington, D.C. 20001
(Demand that the restaurant association ban the use of sulfites in their member establishments.)

Contact your local Health Department officials and bring their attention to this very important issue. Thus far, Texas and California have insisted that restaurants place conspicuous signs stating the use of the chemical. In addition, Pima County in Arizona has banned the use of sulfites, and Chicago is considering a similar resolution. You can help make a difference!

Bibliography

Adams, Ruth and Murray, Frank, *Improving Your Health with Vitamin A*, Larchmont Books, NY, 1978.

Adams, Ruth and Murray, Frank, *Improving Your Health with Vitamin C*, Larchmont Books, NY, 1978.

Adams, Ruth and Murray, Frank, *Improving Your Health with Vitamin E*, Larchmont Books, NY, 1978.

Anderson, John W., *Sulphur in Biology*, Edward Arnold Limited, London, 1978.

Ballentine, Rudolph, M.D., *Diet and Nutrition: A Holistic Approach*, The Himalayan International Institute, Homesdale, PA, 1978.

Blanc, Albert D.G., *So You Have Asthma!*, Charles-C. Thomas Publishers, Springfield, 1966.

Bloomfield, Harold H., M.D. et al, *TM: Discovering Inner Energy and Overcoming Stress*, Delacorte Press, NY, 1975.

Bottomley, H.W., *Allergy: Its Treatment and Care*, Funk and Wagnalls, NY, 1968.

Chapin, Joshua Bicknell, *Asthma, Its Causes and Treatment*, Thomas H. Webb and Co., Boston, 1843.

Hirschfeld, Herman, M.D., F.A.C.A., *The Whole Truth about Allergy*, Arco Publishing Co., NY, 1972.

Indianapolis Technical Societies, *Complying with Sulfur Dioxide Regulations*, Noyes Data Corporation, Park Ridge, NJ, 1972.

Institute of Food Technologists Expert Panel on Food Safety and Nutrition and the Committee on Public Information, "Sulfites and Food Additives," Institute of Food Technologists, Chicago, 1975.

Jacobson, Michael F., *Chemical Additives in Booze*, Center for Science in the Public Interest, Washington, D.C., 1982.

Life Sciences Research Office, "Evaluation of the Health Aspects of Sulfiting Agents as Food Ingredients," Federation of American Societies for Experimental Biology, Bethesda, Maryland, 1976.

Nriagu, Jerome O., *Sulfur in the Environment: Pt. I, The Atmospheric Cycle*, John Wiley and Sons, NY, 1978.

Nriagu, Jerome O., *Sulfur in the Environment: Pt. II, Ecological Impacts*, John Wiley and Sons, NY, 1978.

Null, Gary and staff, *Body Pollution*, Arco Publishing Co., NY, 1973.

Randolph, Theron, M.D., and Moss, Ralph W., PhD., *An Alternate Approach to Allergies*, Bantam Books, NY, 1982.

Rapaport, Howard G., M.D., and Linde, Shirley Motter, M.S., *The Complete Allergy Guide*, Simon and Schuster, NY, 1970.

Rapp, Doris J., M.D., *Allergies and Your Family*, Sterling Publishing Co., NY, 1980.

Rowe, Albert Jr., M.D., *Food Allergy: Its Manifestations and Control and the Elimination Diets*, The Holmes Book Co., Oakland, CA, 1976.

Rudolph, Jack A., M.D., and Rudolph, Burton, M.D., *Victory over Allergies*, Groton Press, Inc., Brooklyn, NY, 1966.

Salter, Henry Hyde, *On Asthma*, Philadelphia, 1864.

Schroeter, Louis C., *Sulfur Dioxide: Applications in Foods, Beverages and Pharmaceuticals*, Permagon Press, Oxford, 1966.

Shriner, David S., et al, *Atmospheric Sulfur Desposition: Environmental Impact and Health Effects*, Ann Arbor Science Publishers, Inc./The Butterworth Group, Ann Arbor, MI, 1980.

Wentzler, Rich, *The Vitamin Book*, St. Martins Press, NY, 1978.

Additional copies of **CANARY IN A COAL MINE** may be ordered by using the order form below:

TO: Aristan Press
Post Office Box 395
Placentia, California 92670

Please send ________ copy (ies) of **CANARY IN A COAL MINE to:**

Name ______________________________

Street Address ______________________________

City, State, Zip ______________________________

I enclose ten dollars ($10) for each copy to cover the cost of the book, postage and handling.

Also available from Aristan Press is the 96-page hardbound edition of **SEND FOR HAYM SALOMON!**, the definitive biography of one of the true unsung heroes of the American Revolution. It can be purchased for $10 postpaid.